Medicinal Herbs

A Beginners Guide to Herbal Medicine for Everyday Health Problems

By

Dermot Farrell

www.healbodymindandspirit.com

MEDICAL DISCLAIMER

The information in this book is not intended to replace professional medical supervision. The information in this book is highly effective and it will definitely reduce the physical and mental health complaints of nearly every person, who earnestly uses the herbs and techniques outlined within. In some cases a cure may take place; however, there is no guarantee that physical ailments will be completely cured. Prior to reducing or stopping allopathic medications, do consult with a qualified physician.

Free Gifts

Bonus #1 – Grab Free Books!!!!!!!!

As a way of saying thank you for downloading this book I would like to give you two free books, which are available exclusively for my readers. The free book "Juicing for Health – 35 Juicing Recipes for Everyday Health Problems", is packed full of useful healthy juice recipes and Success Hacks - 31 Mind-Set Hacks to Increase Productivity and Career Success, is packed full of helpful mind hacks for developing a more dynamic and enjoyable lifestyle!

Please go to my blog page and sign up here:

www.healbodymindandspirit.com

You will receive the two free eBooks, plus weekly updates and even free eBooks!

Bonus#2 - Bonus Video Series

You can check out my YouTube channel, which has lots of health related videos

Please copy the following link into your browser, to access an introduction to herbal remedies video. If you then go to my channel and click playlists, you will find lots of videos on herbs for health:

http://y2u.be/rWpgVltW4dw

If you find it too awkward to type in this code, then you can also find my channel by typing in **www.healbodymindandspirit.com** into the YouTube search

Contents

This book 'Medical Herbs: A Detailed Overview of The Top Herbs for Everyday Health Problems", is the third in a series of books which focuses on to treating everyday health conditions. The first book "Herbs for Depression and Anxiety" focused upon treating mental – emotional health issues via herbal remedies. The second book "Herbal Medicine" focused upon treating 11 chronic health conditions with a wide variety of herbs. This book provides a detailed overview of 8 specific herbs and the idea behind this book is to demonstrate to you the reader how these specific herbs can greatly help you with your everyday health problems.

The first book in the series addresses the reality that 5% of the world's population suffers from some form of clinical depression, at any point in time and that herbs can be used to help relieve the symptoms. The second book provided a wide range of effective herbs and herbal recipes, such as teas and tinctures, which can be used to address a wide variety of everyday health problems. In this the third book in the series, the emphasize is to take the 8 most potent everyday herbs and give a detailed overview about the qualities of these herbs, the benefits of these herbs as well as the way in which they can be used to relieve many everyday health problems.

As a Traditional Chinese Medical Practitioner (TCM practitioner), I have used herbs for many years to great effect and have come to the conclusion that there should be no competition between herbs and allopathic medications. Many allopathic doctors are against herbal treatments and many complementary therapists are against allopathic medications. In my opinion both viewpoints are short sighted. As human beings we have to balance our health and everything which we can leverage in our arsenal, in order to deal with chronic health problems, in order to overcome them. I feel that pharmaceutical medications can be combined with herbal treatments, to the best advantage of the patient. In some cases pharmaceutical drugs can be substituted with herbs, while in other cases herbs can be used in conjunction with pharmaceuticals. The idea is to broaden our portfolio of medicinal health resources, so that we are better prepared to deal with whichever health condition which we may come across, either in our own health or that of our family and friends.

Also, herbs tend to be seen as somewhat mysterious and as something which one uses under the guidance of an experienced complementary therapist. However, I want to address this erroneous idea in his book, as many of the greatest herbs for your health are found within your own kitchen!

As a matter of fact you are eating some of them every day!

In this book we shall explore these herbs and take a detailed look at us how powerful they are and also in many cases we shall see how many of these herbs are quite common and can be used without any expert supervision.

In this the final book, in this series, I hope to spur you on towards understanding and using these herbs in your everyday life, both for your treating chronic everyday health conditions and also they can be used for prevention of ill health!

Yours in health

Dermot Farrell

BA Dip Acu Tcm

Ps

Please check out the other two books in this herbal series (both of which are available on www.amazon.com):

Herbal Medicine (ISBN-10: 1537601245/**ISBN-13:** 978-1537601243)
Herbs for Depression and Anxiety (ISBN-10: 1537601245/ **ISBN-10:** 1537601245)

A Note on Using Herbs

There is a lot of misunderstanding which takes place when people think about using herbs for the relief of chronic health problems. Often people start taking a herb because somebody recommended it to them, only to find out that the herb is apparently useless and of no help to them. Once they reach this conclusion, they promptly stop taking the herb and curse themselves for wasting time and energy with this phoney baloney herb stuff!

However, in many cases herbs proof ineffective because the person has not taken the herb for a long enough period of time, or they are taking an insufficient amount of the herb, or they are not taking the herb frequently enough.

The thing to remember with herbs is that they are not pharmaceutical drugs. On a molecular level pharmaceutical drugs are big molecules which make an immediate and pronounced effect upon the biochemistry of the body. Whereas herbs possess naturally occurring compounds, which at the molecular level are far less pronounced, in their effect.

There are pros and cons to both sides.

9

On a positive side pharmaceutical drugs are very powerful and near immediate in their action, whereas herbs are slow to work and often their action is weak. However drugs have a downside, which is that they produce a lot of side effects, because of the very fact that they produce a profound effect upon the body!

Here the herbs come into their own, because being much milder in action, possessing less efficacy and taking longer to work, herbs are far milder in their effects and they tend to produce far less side effects than drugs.

Now you might ask yourself that if drugs are so powerful, when compared to herbs, then why bother using the herbs at all?

Initially we can counter this argument with the logic that herbs have fewer side effects, but also we can go deeper into this subject. Not only do herbs produce fewer side effects, but also herbs are usually tonic like in their activity, in that they tend to boost the immune system and the overall functioning of the health of the body. We see this, for example, in herbs which assist diabetic care, which not only help to reduce diabetic symptoms but also they reduce the long-term chronic health side effects, which occur in tandem with diabetes, such as heart and circulatory problems, nerve damage and retinopathy of the eyes.

10

This is something which you won't see with drugs. Furthermore with pharmaceuticals, over time, they tend to have a toxic effect upon the body and often, if taken over a long period of time, they will result in organic damage to the body, thus resulting in the need to take on more drugs, to deal with the symptoms caused by the drugs which have been prescribed earlier!

On the other hand, if we combine herbs we tend to get a synergistic effect, whereby one herb boosts the effect of another herb, which is good for our health!

Finally, herbs are not just good at treating ill health, but also they are great preventatives. We must always remind ourselves to try and prevent chronic disease from setting in, as it is far easier to prevent rather than to cure disease!

How to Use Herbs Effectively

The key to using herbs effectively is to first of all realise that herbs take time to work. While most allopathic medications will be working within several hours, herbs will take several days to work and in some cases full efficacy will only come after a couple of weeks of treatment.

So when using herbs don't expect overnight results!

A second consideration with herbs, is that they are generally weaker in action than allopathic medications and consequently you will probably have to combine two or three herbs to produce a significant effect. So rarely will one herb be enough and also the dosage, in some cases, has to be quite big. A popular herb like garlic, for instance, is very effective but you have to take a few grams a day, ideally!

Also on a good note this combination of herbs will actually have a health boosting effect!

Finally frequency is another issue, herbs have to be taken daily and in many cases multiple times a day!

So if you want to get a good result out of herbs, then you have to stop thinking in terms of popping a pill once a day. Herbs don't work that way, they are natural compounds and usually require more frequency, greater dosage and combining one or more herbs at the same time, plus they require a week or two to really start working!

Why Use Both Herbs and Allopathic Medications?

I alluded to this earlier in the foreword: why use both allopathic medications and herbs?

We use both of them because each is a resource. Personally I have grown tired of watching allopathic doctors and complementary therapists fighting each other. As the old saying goes "doctors differ and patients die!" Why are we fighting each other and why are we suggesting that our patients only stick to either drugs or herbs!

Both drugs and herbs are resources and both have their pros and cons. Use them, don't abuse them that's the way to go!

Ideally we should try to substitute allopathic medications for herbs, because herbs have far fewer side effects and can be used over the long-term, often with little or no ill effect. However, the reality of the situation is that many people will not be able to give up allopathic medication. What are you to do if you use multiple herbs, at reasonable dosages and on a daily basis, and yet your chronic health condition either doesn't improve or only improves slightly!

We have to be pragmatic!

While I much prefer to use herbs, sometimes they just don't work as every person has a unique biochemistry.

Another thing to realise is that often whether we are using allopathic medications or herbal medications, we are only treating the symptom and this is an important point. Herbs have wonderful effects upon our health and often they will cure our health problems. But many times herbs will simply relieve our symptoms, just like allopathic medications. Allopathic medications do not cure chronic health conditions, rather they just reduce the intensity of the symptoms and the potential organic damage. Blood pressure medications, for example, balances blood pressure levels which prevents the uncomfortable symptoms of high blood pressure from coming about, but also it prevents organic damage, by maintaining a balanced blood pressure level, which helps to preserve cardiac and kidney health.

Anyway we have to take a pragmatic approach, to using either herbs or allopathic medications, to treat certain health conditions. So while we would like to stop taking allopathic medications altogether, in some case either drugs or herbs are simply part of our treatment plan and as such we should use them in the most effective manner possible.

So, for example, we should try and stop taking drugs, but if that doesn't work, at least we can reduce our dependency on the drugs and reduce the dosage, which will minimise side effects and also help to prevent long-term organic damage. So this is one way in which herbs can be of a great benefit. For many people, who have chronic conditions such as diabetes, high blood pressure and depressive symptoms, for example, may find it impossible to give up allopathic medications and in these cases the herbs will simply assist by allowing for a reduction in dosing!

Finally as noted earlier, sometimes herbs don't work. While I love complementary medicine, I do feel that it is each person's individual responsibility to monitor their health and make sure that they are looking after their health. So while we may like to give up allopathic medications, our first requirement is to maintain the overall balance of our health!

How to Use the Herbs Mentioned in This Book

The herbs which follow are by and large simple and safe in nature, so the easiest thing would be to ignore them. Now just because a herb is popular and widely available doesn't mean that it has to useless!

Each of these top 8 herbs are highly effective, but do follow the advice which has already been laid out. In each chapter detailed information about their many benefits, has been added as well as a variety of recipes, so simply read the information in each chapter and follow the instructions.

Aldo there is a useful appendix, which presents a very helpful table which outlines what health condition each herbs can be used for. So with the appendix you simply have a quick look at each herb and see if it can work on your health problem. For example, garlic is highly effective at treating osteoarthritic conditions. So rather than having to read each chapter in detail, you can always take a look at your symptoms and then refer back to the requisite chapter.

Finally do try out more than one herb. Herbs tend to be weaker in action than pharmaceutical medications, so usually the most effective approach is to try several herbs and use them alongside the allopathic medications. As symptoms improve then start reducing the allopathic medications. Reduce where possible and in some case you can stop taking allopathic medications altogether.

In certain cases the herbs can also be stopped after a while as often the herbs will actually cure the health problem, but in some cases the herbs have simply substituted the allopathic medications, in which case you will have to keep up the herbs. Also on long-term chronic conditions, such as diabetes, these herbs will usually not cure the diabetes, but they will cure the symptoms and prevent most of the long-term organic damage from occurring, so the herbs should be used for life, in this situation. And this is a very important point, in that nobody dies from diabetes, rather they die from the complications of diabetes, and herbs can really help to prevent most of these complications!

So please don't underestimate the herbs but take a mature approach. Also finally consider taking some time out to go and visit with complementary therapists. As a TCM practitioner I can confidently tell you that all health problems are a direct consequences of energetic imbalances, within the body and while we cannot cure every health condition under the sun, in many case herbs combined with complementary therapy works very well and the likelihood of curing your chronic health conditions, will improve a lot when you combine allopathy, herbs, complementary therapies and lifestyle changes, so please keep that in mind!

Part One – 4 Super Foods in Your Kitchen Which May Save Your Life!

Every kitchen has them and everyone uses them, often on a daily or near daily basis, and yet few people realise the awesome medicinal benefit of these 4 herbs which are:

- Honey

- Ginger

- Garlic

- Lemon

If you look around the internet, you will find a lot of useful information about these 4 herbs, but it only really dawned on me, when I wrote my previous book "Herbal Medicine" just how often these 4 herbs keep on popping up, in all kinds of herbal recipes!

I have since concluded that these 4 herbs are both equally good as preventatives as well as being great remedies. I have also come to the conclusion that just about every person on the planet, whether healthy or sick, should be taking either one or more of these herbs, at any given time.

18

Now before going more deeply into the beneficial effects of each of these herbs, we must first begin by overcoming the obvious objection which is "I take these compounds every day and yet my health is no better!" Well if you haven't had a chance to take a look at the introduction, where we outlined how to take these herbs, then do so now. Basically herbs tend to be weaker than drugs and so you have to take:

- A great dosage of herbs
- Frequently (as in every day)
- Several herbs together

In order to get the same benefit as allopathic medications, also the herbs take longer to work.

So while most of us eat garlic and ginger, take lemon in our tea and honey, we do so either infrequently or in a very low dosage. To get the benefit, which these herbs have to offer, you are going to have to take several grams a day, of at least two or more of these herbs, over a period of weeks, in order to see good results.

While these herbs are very popular, to get the best out of them you have to make a point of taking them in sufficient quantity and on a daily basis!

Hopefully with that objection out of the way, we can now take a look at the powerful medicinal benefits of each of these herbs!

Chapter One – Honey

Honey is used in just about every home, mainly because it's tasty, but also it's really healthy, with the following benefits:

· Honey reduces respiratory irritation and coughing frequency and intensity

· It's a strong antibacterial agent

· It's a strong anti-fungal agent

· A strong antiviral

· Can help to improve blood sugar levels, which can help diabetics

· Honey is also a better sugar to take for diabetics than regular refined sugar

· It helps young children sleep

· It's good for eye health

· It's good for cuts

· It's good for burns

Honey reduces Respiratory Irritation and Coughing Frequency and Intensity - Honey Helps Young Children Sleep

Honey is fairly famous as a way to treat sore throats and coughs (both the chesty cough and the dry throaty cough). Most people instinctively realise that honey is nice on your throat, but what most people do not know is that honey is a really strong anti-bacterial agent, which mean that when we take honey, and it drips down our throat, it is effectively killing of the bacteria as it goes. And remember that unlike gargling with an antibiotic agent, honey goes all the way down your throat and oesophagus (passing the opening to the lungs in the process) and down into the stomach. So it's killing bacteria in a very thorough way.

In particular, I feel that honey is very useful for coughs because the standard treatment is to take cough medicine, which although it reduces the irritation; the effect is very short lived because cough medicine is to not very thick, whereas honey possesses a thick viscosity. So when you imbibe honey, without diluting it in any way, the honey slowly drips down your throat, thus giving relief for a long period of time. And another advantage of honey is that you can take as much as you want to, unlike cough medications, which effectively drugs you up if you take too much!

Finally, honey is a really great throat and cough treatment, just before going to bed at night, because the thick viscous liquid, which it is, will provide soothing relief for a good 30 minutes or so, which will help you to relax and get some sleep.

I'm not saying don't take throat and cough medications, but let's be honest when you have a very sore throat or bad cough, no amount of medication is enough. So just remember, next time to reach for that bottle of honey sitting over there in your kitchen cupboard, as it will bring some real relief for cough and sore throats symptoms!

Another helpful use of honey is helping young children to sleep. This will work particular well if they have a cough or sore throat, but even without that say a child who is a little hyper- active or possibly its mid-summer, in the northern or southern hemisphere, and it is till bright until 9pm at night, well in this case give your child some honey before going to bed, as it is a well-known cure for child insomnia!

It's a Strong Antibacterial Agent - It's a Strong Anti-Fungal Agent – It's Good for Cuts and Burns – A Strong Antiviral

We mentioned earlier that honey is a strong antibacterial/antifungal agent, well to prove this some researchers compared the action of honey to antibiotics on four different types of bacteria, which are Pneumococci;

23

Klebsiella Pneumoniae; Pseudomonas Aeruginosa and Staplylococcus Aureus. These are the four most potent chest and throat bacteria and when compared against regular antibiotics the researchers discovered that honey was as effective as the antibiotic at fighting these infections! 1

Meanwhile other research on the common causes of food poisoning - Salmonella, Shigella, Escherichia coli 2 and with the common intestinal bacterial infection Helicobacter pylori 3, have also proven honey to be quite effective. In particular regular imbibing of honey has been shown to protect the gut from infection, by killing of the bacteria which normally adheres to the epithelial cells.4

Of course we must also bear in mind that an antibiotic will circulate around the bloodstream, fighting off infection, whereas honey will only fight infection at a local level, but still it's an impressive finding.

And it doesn't stop there – In another piece of research, this time on treating open leg ulcers, which proved non receptive to regular antibiotics, in a study of 59 patients, 58 out of the 59 made a complete recovery simply by applying honey!5

Honey also works well on burns, if applied to a minor burn it can speed up recovery and if you have any fungal infections imbibing honey, on a daily basis, can also help to bring about relief from symptoms. Honey appears to reduce both the fungal activity and the bacterial activity which improves fungal condition 6, which in turn makes it an effective treatment for such conditions as ringworm and athletes foot!

Honey has also been proven (7) to be an effective treatment for many viruses' and is particular effective at treating herpes virus and rubella virus.7, 8

It's Good for Eye Health

Honey can also be used to treat eye conditions such as corneal injuries, conjunctivitis, keratis, chemical burns to the eyes and thermal burns to the eyes.9,10

Honey is Good for Diabetes

While honey will not cure diabetes, it does help to reduce blood lipids, C-Reactive protein (CRP) levels and homocysteince levels, in both normal as well as diabetic patients.11 Now to put this into perspective, diabetic patients are prone to developing cardiovascular problems and the above coronary markers are strong indicators of potential inflammation and damage to the cardiovascular system. So honey is a really simply way to protect heart health, which is particularly useful for diabetics, but also it's a great help to all of us!

A second positive factor with honey, is that although honey is a sugar, it's not a simple sugar. Rather honey is made from around 40% fructose, 30% glucose, and 10% is constituted from other sugars. Now when compared against both regular refined sugar and glucose, in clinical conditions, honey demonstrated the lowest sugar spike, suggesting that if you want to take a honey for sweetness then honey is far better than regular sugar. 12

Honey for Heart Health

Honey has many properties, which are good for heart health. For a start as noted above, honey helps to reduce common cardiac markers. 11 Also honey is high in phenols, which have anti-ischemic, antithrombotic, anti-oxidant properties, and it also has vasorelaxant properties. In layman's terms this means that honey can protect our heart and also possibly help to reduce blood pressure levels.13 Finally honey is high in nitrous oxide (NO) and this also appears it help to protect heart health. 13

Honey from Traditional Chinese Medical Perspective

My background is in Chinese medicine, so it's interesting to take a look at honey from a Chinese medical perspective.

Form a TCM point of view, honey is neutral and sweet in nature which makes it capable of nourishing and lubricating the inner organs, particularly the lungs. Honey boosts the functioning of the stomach and spleen (energetic channels), it improves appetite, boosts energy levels and reduces pain. It detoxifies the body, reduces internal heat within the body, which has a nurturing effect.

So from a TCM perspective honey is a tonic, in the old fashioned sense as a compound which picks you up and rebuilds your health.

Final Thoughts on Honey and How to Take It

Hopefully after reading this section, you have come to see that good old honey is a far more potent medicine, than you ever thought possible. As I already stated, at the beginning of this chapter, I too was kind of oblivious to honey until I wrote my earlier book "herbal medicine". So just because honey is common doesn't mean it doesn't work.

As we can see honey is so effective, that not only can it cure many conditions but also it is a great health preventative. Its effect on C -

Reactive protein, homocysteince and blood lipids alone should be enough to encourage you to take honey everyday, for the rest of your life!

Finally How to Take Honey?

Apart from external treatments, where you apply honey externally to a wound or a burn, honey is simply imbibed by mouth. You can take it directly from the jar, around one or two tablespoons per day is enough to produce a good effect, ideally once in the morning and once in the evening. Also, you can take honey with your tea or coffee instead of sugar, as a sweetener. It mixes well in juices and smoothies and it is fantastically tasty, when mixed in with muesli and can also be mixed successfully (although fattening, with peanut butter and protein powder!)

But the one final thing to note here, is that most honey, which you find on your supermarket shelves, is good but it's not very pure. Ideally you should go for the best honey, which you can get. The most pure version is organic honeycomb, which tastes amazing and which will turbocharge your energy levels, however, it's very expensive and this is a factor to bear in mind with honey. Remember to get a benefit out of honey, you're looking at taking about two tablespoons a day, which is about 30grams a day. So this could become expensive, if you are using a top of the range honey. Also some honeys are expensive but not very good. As a rule of thumb, the darker the better, so buy honey according to your budget. Try to avoid very low quality ones, but also accept that unless you're wealthy, the highest quality honey will probably not be within your budget!

Footnotes

1.   ANTIBACTERIAL ACTIVITY OF HONEY AGAINST BACTERIA ISOLATED FROM RESPIRATORY TRACT INFECTIONS

Farhan Essaa Abdullah, Kiran Afab, Rabia Khanum, Sidrah Sohail Khan

Journal of Dow University of Health Science (JDUHS) Vol 6, No 3 (2012) > Abdullah

2.   Alvarez-Suarez JM, Tulipani S, Romandini S, Bertoli E, Battino M. Contribution of honey in nutrition and human health: a review. Mediterr J Nutr Metab. 2010;3:15–23.

3.   Chowdhury M. Honey: is it worth rubbing it in? J Rl Soc Med. 1999;92:663–664

4.   Alnaqdy A, Al-Jabri A, Al Mahrooqi Z, Nzeako B, Nsanze H. Inhibition effect of honey on the adherence of Salmonella to intestinal epithelial cells in vitro. Int J Food Microbiol. 2005;103:347–351.

5.   Clinical observations on the wound healing properties of honey

Mr. S. E. E. Efem*

Article first published online: 8 DEC 2005

DOI: 10.1002/bjs.1800750718

6.   Bansal V, Medhi B, Pandhi P. Honey -A remedy rediscovered and its therapeutic utility. Kathmandu Univ Med J. 2005;3:305–309

7.   Al-Waili NS. Investigating the antimicrobial activity of natural honey and its effects on the pathogenic bacterial infections of surgical wounds and conjunctiva. J Med Food . 2004;7:210–222.

8.   Al-Waili NS, Haq A. Effect of honey on antibody production against thymus-dependent and thymus-independent antigens in primary and secondary immune responses. J Med Food. 2004;7:491–494.

9.   Meda A, Lamien EC, Millogo J, Romito M, Nacoulma OG. Ethnopharmacological communication therapeutic uses of honey and honeybee larvae in central Burkina Faso. J Ethnopharmacol. 2004;95:103–107.

10.   Shenoy R, Bialasiewicz A, Khandekar R, Al Barwani B, Al Belushi H. Traditional medicine in Oman. its role in ophthalmology. Middle East Afr J Ophthalmol. 2009;16:92–96

11.   Al-Waili NS. Natural honey lowers plasma glucose, c-reactive protein, homocysteine, and blood lipids in healthy, diabetic, and hyperlipidemic subjects: comparison with dextrose and sucrose. J Med Food. 2004;7:100–107.

12.   Plasma Glucose Responses to Glucose, Sucrose, and Honey in Patients with Diabetes Mellitus: An Analysis of Glycaemic and Peak Incremental Indices

Samanta, A. C. Burden andA. R. Jones Senior Medical Registrar*

Article first published online: 30 JUL 2009

DOI: 10.1111/j.1464-5491.1985.tb00654.x

1985 Diabetes UK

13.   Khalil MI, Sulaiman SA. The potential role of honey and its polyphenols in preventing heart diseases: a review. Afr J Tradit Complement Altern Med . 2010;7:315–321

Chapter Two - Ginger

Ginger is very popular as an ingredient in many tasty recipes, but what most people do not know is that ginger is a fantastic tonic which has the following benefits:

· Ginger strengthens the immune system

· Ginger cures nausea

· Ginger reduces high blood pressure

· Ginger helps to reduce the severity of symptoms associated with osteoarthritis

· Ginger helps to reduce blood sugar levels in diabetics

· Ginger improves digestion

· Ginger reduces bad cholesterol

· Ginger prevents dementia

· Ginger reduces the symptoms of menstrual tension

· Ginger boosts yang energy in the body

· Ginger is a great tonic

Ginger Strengthens the Immune System

Ginger possesses amazing antiseptic, anti-inflammatory and antiviral properties. Ginger is also a chest decongestant, a natural antihistamine, a milder sedative and a natural pain killer!

All of these benefits comes about because ginger is high in sesquiterpenes, which are a naturally occurring compound which have amazing immune system boosting properties, and have been proven clinically as a cure for rhinovirus, so next time you will a runny nose coming on then consider taking ginger on a regular basis![1]

Ginger Cures Nausea

Ginger is a really great way to cure symptoms of nausea. If you are feeling nausea, then simply take a few slices of ginger root crush them a little bit and then add to water, boil and then leave to simmer for 5 minutes, strain and serve!

Does ginger really work on nauseas?

Yes it does and it has been clinically proven to do so. In a study on ladies suffering from morning sickness, they gave them 1 gram of ginger per day and 28 out of the 32 participants found a noticeable relief from symptoms of morning sickness!2

Ginger Reduces High Blood Pressure

High blood pressure is up in the top 10 list of most deadly conditions according to the World Health Organisation (WHO). The problem with high blood pressure is that it increases the build-up of plaque in the arteries and it promotes heart and kidney damage, which over time can increase the risk of heart failure, heart attacks and strokes, so anything which reduces high blood pressure is a good thing!

Anyway in clinical trials with ginger they have seen a drop in blood pressure of approximately 10%, so someone who has a blood pressure level of 140 over 90 (which is borderline high) will end up in the low 130's over low 80's which is very good!3

Ginger Helps to Reduce the Severity of Symptoms Associated with Osteoarthritis

Osteoarthritis is a painful joint condition which negatively impacts tens of millions of people all over the world today. In clinical trials on 247

34

participants, who suffered from osteoarthritic knee pain, they noted a significant reduction in symptoms by the end of the six week trial. 4

Ginger Helps to Reduce Blood Sugar Levels in Diabetics

Like high blood pressure diabetes is in the WHO top 10 of most hazardous diseases. Not that anyone dies from diabetes, but rather they die from complications, which have come about via the long-term degenerative effects of diabetics. So needless to say anything which improves diabetic health is a good thing and the most important factor relating to diabetes is to reduce blood sugar levels. Ginger has been studied and in one trial of 41 participants they noted that over a course of a 12 week period, while taking 2 grams of ginger a day, that the overall average fasting blood sugar levels dropped by 12%. 5

This means that a person who has say a borderline diabetic blood sugar level of 140mgdl (7.7 mmol), could see a reduction back down to 125mgdl(6.9mmol), ok not perfect but a lot better for your long-term health than 140/7.7!

Ginger Improves Digestion

Digestion begins with the stomach and ends with the intestines. The purpose of the stomach is to quickly break down the food into a syrup, which can easily travel through the small intestines. When this process slows down, it results in a feeling of heaviness and indigestion.

Ginger, as it happens, is a great way to treat indigestion. In a study of 24 participants, they noted that those who took 1.2grams of ginger, one hour before their meal, emptied the contents of their stomach twice as quickly as those who didn't take the ginger. On average the control group took 27 minutes, whereas the ginger taking group took just 13 minutes, to empty their stomachs.6

Now you might be thinking was has the speed of time it takes to empty one's stomach got to do with digestion?

Well the thing to remember, is that if the food is emptying from the stomach at a far faster rate, then it must be digesting faster, which in turn means that the intestines are getting fully liquefied food. One of the problems with indigestion and bloatedness, is that the food does not digest well, in the stomach, and instead semi-solid food enters the intestines and takes a long time to process.

So this clinical trial suggests that we should all probably take some ginger prior to a heavy meal, like when we go out to dinner for example, it will really help to avoid bloatedness. Also for people who are prone to slow digestion, indigestion and acid reflux, taking ginger either before or with meals is probably a good idea.

Ginger Reduces Bad Cholesterol

We have all heard about the pitfalls of cholesterol (or should we say bad cholesterol as some cholesterol is good for health). Anyway LDL, VLDL cholesterol and triglycerides are the bad cholesterol, and when high they can result in the build-up of harmful plaque in the arteries. Arterial plaque is a lot like the plaque on our teeth, in that it is a thick hard substance, which builds up and in the case of arteries they end up getting blocked because of this plaque.

The obvious way to avoid high levels of bad cholesterol is to eat a healthy diet with low saturated fat levels and also to exercise. But in some case, due to personal genetics, some people are prone to high cholesterol levels, even when they do all the right things.

In a study on 85 participants, who took 3 grams of ginger per day, for a 45 days period, they saw a significant reduction in triglycerides, and very low density lipoprotein (VLDL) levels low density lipoprotein (LDL).7

So if you have high cholesterol levels or just want to keep them at bay then get started with ginger today!

Ginger Prevents Dementia

Dementia, the breaking down of the brain in old people resulting in memory lapses and confusion, is extremely common in the elderly, however here again ginger can help. Ginger appears to work well as an anti-inflammatory in the body and in tests promising results demonstrate that the anti-inflammatory properties of ginger may help to stop the onset of dementia in older people. Research so far is not conclusive but clinical trials on the chemical mechanism at work suggests that the ginger may preserve brain health by reducing inflammation, which helps to maintain the effective functioning of the brain.8

Ginger Reduces the Symptoms of Pre-Menstrual Tension

Noting what was just said in the last section on dementia, ginger reduces inflammation and this is really helpful for ladies, who are suffering from Pre-Menstrual Tension (PMT). In a study, where they took 150 women and gave them 1 gram of ginger per day, for the first three days of the menstrual period, they noted in this study that taking just 1 gram of ginger per day, was equally effective as taking either 400mg of ibuprofen or 250mg of mefanamic acid 4 times a day!9

So for ladies who are suffering from PMT, they can either take ginger instead of pain killers or in the case of ladies who suffer severe PMT cramping symptoms, then the two could be combined effectively for greater relief!

Ginger Boosts Yang Energy in the Body

Image As a Traditional Chinese Medical practitioner I have to mention that ginger is high in yang energy (active energy). The energy of the body is a balance between yang and ying energy:

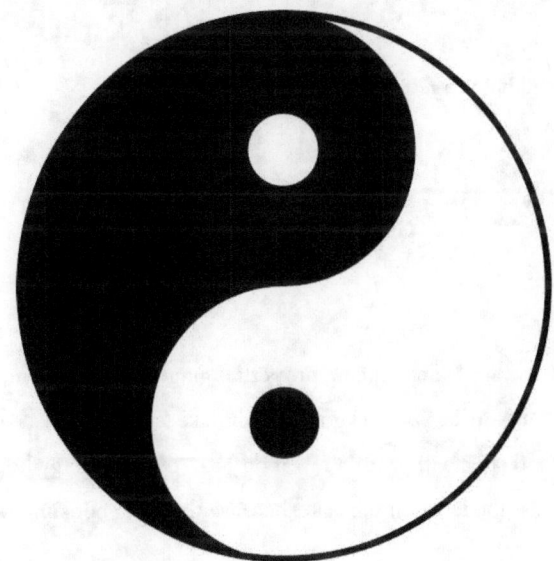

Yang	Ying
Active	Passive
Male	Female
Invigorating	Nurturing

So everything in the body is a balance between these two energies. Too little ying energy and a person will feel anxious, desperate and paranoid. Too little yang energy and a person will feel flat, lazy and lacklustre. As a rule of thumb most people on this planet lack yang energy and they do so because we are too busy (not resting enough), we don't recharge our batteries (not enough rest and sleep), we think too much (too much thinking burns off spleen yang Qi (CHI) energy) and we have a poor diet!

So ginger will help to rebalance this energetic imbalance.

Ginger is a Great Tonic

Because of its yang Qi enhancing properties ginger is a great tonic. It will pick you up and make you feel good, if you take 2 or 4 grams a day on a daily basis and stick with it for a few months. Now the energy boosting effects are just the icing on the cake, because this yang boosting herb will

40

help, over time, right the energetic imbalance which could be causing some health problems such as diabetes, high blood pressure, painful haemorrhoids, headaches, insomnia and so on.

For example, at one time my resting heart rate was a little on the low side (in the 40's bpm), after taking ginger on a daily basis for a few months, my resting heart rate moved up into the 50's bpm. In theory having a very low resting heart rate is good, if you are an elite athlete with a very healthy heart. However, although I go to the gym 5 or 6 days a week, I am not an athlete, so my heart rate should be higher. Back in my youth my resting heart rate was around 60bpm, so this is probably ideal for me. Anyway moving up from high 40's to low mid 50's is step in the right direction and this is all thanks to taking ginger!

So the funny thing with taking ginger on a regular basis, is that if you stick with it for a few months, you shall see some quirky improvement in one or more health parameters. Ginger been an herb, its effects are gentle and slow to work, so don't expect anything amazing, but over time it will really help your health.

Another thing which I noted over many years of treating patients with TCM, I often noted that from session to session that my patients would report no great difference between sessions, but then when I asked them about symptoms, they would note that many of them had disappeared!

The conversation would usually go like this:

Dermot:	"Hi any difference from last week?"
Patient:	"No pretty much the same"
Dermot:	"How are the headaches?"
Patient:	"Definitely a little better"
Dermot:	"And sleep?"
Patient:	"Yeah, I've got good sleep most of this week"
Dermot:	"How about the indigestion?"
Patient:	"Yeah that too it's a bit better, come to think of it, it's a lot better"

So I discovered that my patients where improving, but with complementary medicine improvement is gradual and often symptoms just disappear, unlike allopathic medications which hit your body like a hammer. This is something to bear in mind not only with TCM but all complementary therapies and indeed herbs too. Don't expect lighting fast changes, rather expect gradual improvement. It's something which we are not used to anymore because we expect fast results, but the results which we get from drugs are not natural and often while a symptom improves, our overall balance of health does not. Remember we are looking for improved overall health and ginger will greatly help in this process if you

42

take enough if it, frequently enough and for a long enough period of time!

The Best Ways to Take Ginger

There are lots of good ways to take ginger supplementation. The easiest way is to take supplements out of a bottle, which is fine, especially since it can be difficult to get enough ginger was raw ginger, is very difficult to take unless you mix it in with a juice or a smoothie. So let's take a look at a few alternatives, as while capsules are fine, raw is always best!

Also regarding dosage around 2 to 3 grams a day is good. If you want to take raw ginger, say in a tea or a juice or a smooth, then it is difficult to know exactly how much you are taking. So as a rule of thumb I would suggest 1 cup or mug of ginger tea for maintenance and 3 cups or mugs a day for anyone who is really drained or removing from chronic ill health.

If you are taking 3 cups a day, of the concentrated "Holistic Super Healthy Ginger Tea" option below then I would recommend only taking this much for 6 weeks at any one time, then take a few weeks at maintenance levels. We have to watch our ying and yang levels, so too much of this herb could burn of nurturing energy at a very high dosage!

Juices and Smoothies: If you want to add ginger into smoothness and juices, it's really easy, simply peel the outer skin from the part of ginger which you intend on taking and then slice off 3 to 5 bits, then throw them in the mix and off you go!

Ginger Tea: Ginger tea is a great option as you can get a real kick out of it. Here are two suggestions:

Traditional Indian Ginger Tea

1.   Mix one cup of milk with one cup of water (this is to make two cups of tea)

2.   Add sugar (if you like sugar) into the mix

3.   Add two teaspoons of tea powder

4.   Add in several slices of ginger (cut and then crush it a little bit so as to get the most out of it)

5.   Boil, simmer and boil simmer gain three times

6.   Strain and serve

Holistic Super Healthy Ginger Tea

1.   Take 2 cups of water (for 2 cups) and add in several slices of ginger (cut and then crush it a little bit so as to get the most out of it)

2.   Boil and leave to simmer for 10 minutes

3.   Squeeze one small lemon or half a medium sized lemon into each cup

4.   Add one to two tablespoons of honey per cup (depending upon taste…ginger tea is very strong so a fair amount of honey is required to take out the sting!)

5.   Strain and pour the ginger water solution into each cup

The advantage with this full blown way to take ginger tea, is that the ginger is so much stronger, because you have let it simmer for a good 10 minutes. So as to know when the concoction is ready, simply waited until the water has taken on a distinct yellowy brown hue.

You can click on this link to see a YouTube video outlining how to make ginger tea. Also it provides a nice detailed outline of the yang/yang theory and how this has an effect on your health!

Please note that the first half of this video outlines the benefits of ginger and the second part shows you how to make the ginger tea.

Anyway the advantage of this concentrated version of ginger tea is that the ginger is very strong, so strong that it should sting your throat a little bit. Also honey and lemon have many great additional benefits.

For general health Indian ginger tea is great, but if you are under the weather and need to pick yourself up or are trying to recover from chronic ill health, then I would suggest going for the more concentrated option!

Contraindications

Ginger is a very safe herb although there are a couple of contraindications.

1.   Ginger slows blood clotting and may adversely affect medications which are designed thin the blood such as 'warfarin'

2.   Ginger reduces blood sugar, to the degree that diabetics should monitor their blood sugar levels, as ginger can cause a pretty severe drop in blood sugar levels in some cases!

3.   Massive doses of concentrated ginger could adversely affect ying energy, but this should not be a problem if you follow the advice given above in the section entitled "The Best Way to Take Ginger"

Footnotes

1.   J Nat Prod. 1994 May;57(5):658-62.

Isolation of antirhinoviral sesquiterpenes from ginger (Zingiber officinale).

Denyer CV, Jackson P, Loakes DM, Ellis MR, Young DA.

2.   Ginger for Nausea and Vomiting in Pregnancy: Randomized, Double-Masked, Placebo-Controlled Trial

VUTYAVANICH, TERAPORN MD, MSC; KRAISARIN, THEERAJANA MD; RUANGSRI, RUNG-AROON BSC.

3.   J Cardiovasc Pharmacol. 2005 Jan;45(1):74-80.

Ginger lowers blood pressure through blockade of voltage-dependent calcium channels.

Ghavur MN, Gilani Ah

4.   Arthritis Rheum. 2001 Nov;44(11):2531-8.

Effects of a ginger extract on knee pain in patients with osteoarthritis.

Altman RD, Marcussen KC.

Miami Veterans Affairs Medical Center and University of Miami, Florida, USA.

5.   Iran J Pharm Res. 2015 Winter; 14(1): 131–140.

PMCID: PMC4277626

The Effects of Ginger on Fasting Blood Sugar, Hemoglobin A1c, Apolipoprotein B, Apolipoprotein A-I and Malondialdehyde in Type 2 Diabetic Patients

Nafiseh Khandouzi,a Farzad Shidfar,b,* Asadollah Rajab,c Tayebeh Rahideh,d Payam Hosseini,e and Mohsen Mir Taherif

6.   Eur J Gastroenterol Hepatol. 2008 May;20(5):436-40. doi: 10.1097/MEG.0b013e3282f4b224.

Effects of ginger on gastric emptying and motility in healthy humans.

Wu KL, Rayner CK, Chuah SK, Changchien CS, Lu SN, Chiu YC, Chiu KW, Lee CM.

7.   Saudi Med J. 2008 Sep;29(9):1280-4.

Investigation of the effect of ginger on the lipid levels. A double blind controlled clinical trial.

Alizadeh-Navaei R, Roozbeh F, Saravi M, Pouramir M, Jalali F, Moghadamnia AA.

8.   Drug Des Devel Ther. 2014; 8: 2045–2059.

Published online 2014 Oct 23. doi: 10.2147/DDDT.S67778

PMCID: PMC4211852

Faizul Azam,Abdualrahman M Amer, Abdullah R Abulifa, and Mustafa M Elzwawi

9.   J Altern Complement Med. 2009 Feb;15(2):129-32. doi: 10.1089/acm.2008.0311.

Comparison of effects of ginger, mefenamic acid, and ibuprofen on pain in women with primary dysmenorrhea.

Ozgoli G, Goli M, Moattar F.

Chapter Three – Garlic

Garlic is a famous ingredient for many wonderfully tasty dishes, and it's fair to say that it is present in most people's kitchens. But like so many wonderful medicinal herbs, it is underrated as an herbal remedy. In reality garlic is one of the most powerful common herbs, which you can find, and it can cure many health conditions which includes the following:

- Garlic reduces cold and flu symptoms

- Garlic reduces blood pressure

- Garlic reduces cholesterol levels

- Garlic helps to protect heart health

- Garlic reduces blood glucose levels

- Garlic can improve Alzheimer symptoms & Prevent the Onset of Dementia

- Garlic detoxifies the body

- Garlic can strengthen bones

- Garlic is an anti-allergen

- Garlic boosts sex hormones?

· Garlic cures cancer!

In the last section we provided an overview of ginger and ginger has an amazing range of benefits. Garlic is another one of those natural tonics, which enhance the vitality of the body, not just relieve symptoms, but actually recharge our health!

Garlic Reduces Cold and Flu Symptoms

In the movies garlic is used to fend of vampires... I can see why! Garlic is a great herb which promotes health and defends the body from ill health and infection!

Garlic is high in vitamins A, B1, B6, C, phosphorous and iron. Most importantly it is high in Allicin, which is an all-round health booster. In clinical trials, they noted a 65% reduction in the onset of cold's and an 80% reduction in intensity of symptoms, using 180mg a day of allicin.[1] Approximately 100mg is found in one clove of garlic.

So if you want to keep away the common cold or reduce the intensity of a cold or flu, once it has taken hold then takes 4 cloves of raw garlic a day.

Another important factor here is that the garlic should be raw. I know a lot of people like garlic in their cooking and certainly cooked garlic will help both the flavour of your food and your overall feeling of health and wellbeing, but once it's cooked it loses some of its potency. So either eat garlic raw or take garlic capsules.

Finally, in case you are wondering whether or not garlic can really prevent the onset of a cold or flu and reduce the intensity of the symptoms, I can provide some anecdotal evidence. Some years ago I was coming down with a severe cold and then a colleague suggested that I take "the scented rose", that is garlic. I bought myself a bulb of garlic and ate all 16 cloves raw and in one go!!!

I don't recommend doing that, as it hurt my stomach; raw garlic is quite acidic when it hits your stomach. Anyway the next day I woke up with no cold!

Ok what I did was extreme but it does go to show that garlic is very powerful. Obviously don't eat a whole bulb raw, but do take some capsules with your meals or take a couple of raw cloves and chop them up and add them to your meals and you will get a very similar benefit!

Garlic Reduces Blood Glucose Levels/Blood Pressure – Reduces Bad Cholesterol – Protects Heart Health

Garlic reduces blood glucose levels.1

Once again we see the beneficial effects of Allicin at work in relieving blood pressure and in promoting cardiac health. In clinical trials garlic has produced a significant drop in blood pressure levels.2

In another study comparing the effects of garlic on 45 participants versus a control group of 40 participants, it resulted in a significant reduction in triglyceride, cholesterol, very low density lipoprotein (VLDL) and low density lipoprotein (LDL) and levels, in comparison to the control group.3

In another study on diabetic rats, garlic oil demonstrated positive heart health effects. 4 Does this mean that garlic is good for human hearts? As of yet the jury is out, but there is a good chance that this is the case.

In summation, these are some of the good results regarding the cardiac/blood pressure/cholesterol health boosting effects of garlic. If you take a look at the research on garlic and cardiovascular health, you will note a wide range of research, some of which suggests that garlic is good and others that it is ineffectual.

One of the challenges, with research into herbs, is that it's far from extensive. Scientists require funding for research and it is far easier to get funding for drugs than for herbs. Hence research on herbs tends to be rare, compared to research on drugs, plus the research tends to be on fairly small sample groups.

So what can we take from this?

I feel that there are enough promising studies to suggest that garlic is good for heart health, but it's not definitive. One thing that does keep on popping up, is the emphasize on raw garlic, in large amounts versus cooked garlic. If you want to get a good effect from garlic definitely you need to take several grams a day either from raw garlic or garlic liquid capsules. Cooked garlic seems to lose most of its potency.

One thing that does keep on popping up, is the emphasize on raw garlic, in large amounts versus cooked garlic!

Allicin, in particular seems to have amazing effects. Here are some of the effects of Allicin:

- Allicin reduces blood pressure levels

- Allicin protects heart health and reduces the onset of strokes, heart attacks and ischemic heart disease

- Allicin reduces cholesterol levels

- Allicin reduces blood glucose levels

- Allicin boosts the potency of the bodies antibodies (which makes for better immunity)

- Allicin is an effective anti-microbial agent

- Allicin can prevent the common cold

- Allicin shows promise as a potential cancer treating agent

So Allicin is quite an amazing compound and it is prominent in garlic. However, while in general each clove of garlic possesses around 2500mcg's of Allicin, it can vary from individual clove to individual clove, plus cooked garlic appears to either possess no Allicin or it is inactive.

Research suggests at least 10000mcg's of Allicin a day (approximately 4 cloves) to have a good effect on health, and some researchers are still not sure if even raw garlic will do the trick. One option is to buy Allicin capsules, as its pure Allicin and this is probably a good idea. Although I would still suggest, taking garlic, because there are other compounds in garlic which also boost health. Pharmaceutical companies often take out one compound from an herb, and present it in a capsule, and although it works usually some other benefits are lost.

Probably the best option is to take Allicin capsules and eat raw garlic whenever possible, that way you are getting the best out of both worlds!

Garlic Can Improve Alzheimer Symptoms & Prevent the Onset of Dementia

In a study on the effects of Aged Garlic Extract (AGE), they noted a significant benefit for "anti-oxidant/anti-inflammatory activities with hypolipidemic, antiplatelet and neuroprotective effects".5

So what does this mean in plain English?

What it basically suggests is that garlic has anti-inflammatory properties, which helps to slow down and even preserve brain cells, from age related damage. While many researchers still question the effects of garlic on cardiovascular health, the research regarding garlics brain boosting effects, appears to be more positive.

If you want to do yourself a health favour then take garlic for your brain health. Also looking back on the last section, garlic and cardiovascular health, we noted that Allicin can work very well as a pill type supplement. But for brain health, it is the other properties of garlic, which appear to promote brain health, so this is a good reason to take raw garlic whenever possible.

Allicin can work very well as a pill type supplement. But for brain health, it is the other properties of garlic, which appear to promote brain health, so this is a good reason to take raw garlic whenever possible!

Finally there is some good news that even brain cancer can be cured via garlic. In a study they noted that three organo-sulphur compounds, which are found in garlic (DAS, DADS, DAT) appear to kill cancer brain cancer cells!6

For brain health take the garlic cloves and remove the skin and let them lie in the open air for 15 minutes prior to cooking!

Apparently the best way to take garlic for brain health, according to Ray Swapan, the author of this study, is to simply cut and peel the garlic 15 minutes prior to cooking it, so as to release the enzyme alliinase, which will unlock the cancer eating organo-sulphur compounds. So great, what a simply way to protect your brain health and gain more benefit from cooked garlic, at the same time!

Cut and peel the garlic cloves and leave them in the air for 15 minutes and then eat them or cook with them, as this will release allianase, which will activate the brain saving compounds from within the garlic!

Garlic Detoxifies the Body

Garlic is also famous for its liver detoxifying properties and clinical research backs up the anecdotal evidence. In one study they noted that the organo-sulphur compounds found in garlic, improved the antioxidant system in liver and blood. 7 And in another study, on lead detoxification in patients, who suffered from "chronic occupational lead poisoning", noted a significant improvement in liver detoxification.8

In this occupational lead poisoning study, 117 car battery workers were randomly grouped into two groups. The first group where given 250mg's of d-penicillamine (an allopathic treatment for hepatoxicity), 3 times daily for 4 weeks and the second group where given 1.2mcg's of Allicin (from approximately 1000mg's of garlic), 3 times daily for 4 weeks. Both groups saw an improvement in hepatoxicity, but the d-penicillamine group had more side effects and the garlic group saw a noticeable reduction in blood pressure levels, headaches symptoms and decreased deep tendon reflex, within the 4 week testing period!

So what can we take from this?

What these two studies, which only represent a small number as there are lots of studies out there, represent a very realistic detoxification potency, which lies with garlic, as a result of the organo-sulphur compounds (the same compounds which fight brain cancer!).

In the first study they focused on the effects of GO, DAS and DAT, whereas in the second study they focused on allicin. All of these are organo-sulphur compounds, so to summarize allicin is having a hepatoxic effect and so are other organo-sulphur compounds. In total garlic contains approximately 33 organo-sulphur compounds, so once again while allicin is great, it's a good idea to eat raw garlic cloves as well, for the extra health benefits, offered by a wide range of organo-sulphur compounds!

Garlic detoxifies the body, this is clinically proven, it's not just another feel good herb, and it really works. Also liver toxicity is a major issue both in some illnesses and also as a consequence of taking some drugs, so anything which can detox the liver is really helpful!

Garlic Can Strengthen Bones

Garlic is also really good for bone health. In a study carried out by Kings College London on 1000 female twins, they noted that ladies eating vegetables which are high in allium, particularly garlic and onions, demonstrated noticeably less osteoarthritis of the hips then those who did not eat vegetables, which are high in allium (Allicin comes from allium).9 And in another study they noted that allium reduces bone reabsorption, which could explain why garlic (and also onions by the way) are good for bone health.10

Bone health is a complex subject and there appear to be many mechanisms, by which herbs can help to strengthen bones. Another bone strengthening benefit for menopausal women, is also found in garlic. In a study carried out on 44 postmenopausal osteoporotic women, which were divided into two groups, a garlic group and a placebo group, they noted that the group who took garlic showed a 47% decreases in TNF-α (tumour necrosis factor), a compound which in elevated amounts has been found to increase cell death and which is part of the bodies inflammation response.11 TNF-α inhibitors are a common treatment option for osteoarthritis, so garlic is producing a similar effect naturally!

Garlic is an Anti-Allergen

60

Garlic is a great way to fight allergies. In a study on the action of garlic, they noted that Aged Garlic Extract (AGE) reduced a significant reduction in mast cells and activated T Lymphocytes, which are instrumental in the histamine response.12

How should we take garlic for allergies?

Garlic can be taken either raw or in capsule form. Take 2 cloves, chop them and add them in with each meal (6 cloves a day over 3 meals), whenever you feel an allergic response stating to come on. Garlic been a natural product will work more slowly than pharmaceutical grade anti-histamine, so when you are caught out by an allergic response do take the anti-histamine and then add in the garlic. For people who are prone to feeling an allergic response, at certain times of the year, then take garlic every day. For example, a lot of people suffer from hay fever in the spring, so in this case make a point of upping your raw garlic or garlic capsule intake as this season approaches.

Take 2 cloves, chop them and add them in with each meal (6 cloves a day over 3 meals), whenever you feel an allergic response stating to come on!

Garlic Boosts Hormone Levels?

There is mixed clinical evidence to support the theory that garlic boosts oestrogen and testosterone levels. However, this research tends to be on rats and while rats might get a boost from garlic, this does not necessarily mean that garlic will work as a hormone boosting therapy in human beings.

The clinical tests on rats show a promising trend, which with more clinical research (this time on humans), might proof that garlic has a potential effect here. While I'm all for herbs versus pharmaceutical intervention, it is unlikely that garlic will make a significant impact on menopausal women or hypogondal men. However, as always it is a good idea for people who are low on sex hormones to take garlic, for the same reason that it is a good idea to take ginger. Both garlic and ginger are strong yang enhancing herbs and they have tonic like effects on the body, but do not expect to reverse impotence simply based on eating garlic alone!

From my experience as a Traditional Chinese Medical Practitioner, I think it likely that in some case where the individual is suffering from a very big energetic deficiency, that herbs such as garlic and ginger might well help restore some degree of hormonal function. Of course, there is no guarantee about this and it will vary from individual to individual.

Garlic Cures Cancer!

There is actually a surprising amount of good evidence which suggests that garlic does indeed cure some cancers. In a study from 2003, on using garlic to treat patients who were suffering with benign hyperplasia and prostate cancer, they gave each patient 1ml of aqueous garlic capsules per kilogram (2.2lbs) of bodyweight. So a man weighing 75 kilograms (165lbs) would take 75ml of aqueous garlic capsules per day. The participants, in this trial demonstrated decreased urination frequency, increased urine volume and decreased prostrate size.13

In another study on lung cancer, 1424 patients and 4543 healthy subjects who attended interviews, where they were asked about their eating habits noticed that a significant number of healthy people appeared to have avoided the onset of lung cancer via their garlic intake!14

Also we already noted earlier in this section that garlic has brain cancer fighting properties, in the section on dementia; see footnote number 6, for more details.

So to sum up garlic, as a cancer preventative and treatment protocol, I'm not suggesting that a cancer patient should drop all medications and eat garlic! Rather I am suggesting that garlic is an herb which has some cancer preventative/cancer healing effects, in the case of some but not all cancers!

Like all the herbs in this book, garlic is an herb which should be a regular part of a healthy lifestyle. The healthier your lifestyle the less likely there will be an imbalance and the more likely you will have good health!

Footnotes

1. Antidiabetic effect of garlic (Allium sativum L.) in normal and streptozotocin-induced diabetic rats

A. Eidi , M. Eidi, E. Esmaeili

Phytomedicine-Volume 13, Issues 9–10, 24 November 2006, Pages 624–629

2.   Can Garlic Lower Blood Pressure? A Pilot Study

F. Gilbert McMahon M.D., Ramon Vargas M.D.

Clinical Research Center, New Orleans, Louisiana.

First published: 8 July 1993

DOI: 10.1002/j.1875-9114.1993.tb02751.x

3.   J Agric Food Chem. 2010 Oct 13;58(19):10347-55. doi: 10.1021/jf101606s.
64

Cardiac contractile dysfunction and apoptosis in streptozotocin-induced diabetic rats are ameliorated by garlic oil supplementation.

Ou HC, Tzang BS, Chang MH, Liu CT, Liu HW, Lii CK, Bau DT, Chao PM, Kuo WW.

4.   Effects of organosulfur compounds from garlic oil on the antioxidation system in rat liver and red blood cells

C.C Wu, L.Y Sheen, H.-W Chen, S.-J Tsai, C.-K Lii,

5.   Proteomic Analysis of the Effects of Aged Garlic Extract and Its FruArg Component on Lipopolysaccharide-Induced Neuroinflammatory Response in Microglial Cells

Mawhinney,2 Paula N. Brown,8 Kevin L. Fritsche,6 Mark Hannink,2 Dennis B. Lubahn,2 Grace Y. Sun,1,2,3 and Zezong Gu1,3,7,

Shawn Hayley, Editor

6.   Antosiewicz J, Ziolkowski W, Kar S, Powolny A.A, Singh S.V. Role of reactive oxygen intermediates in cellular responses to dietary cancer chemopreventive agents. Planta Med. 2008;74:1570–9.

Accepted 20 November 2000, Available online 15 May 2001

7.   Saudi Pharm J. 2010 Jan; 18(1): 51–58.

Published online 2009 Dec 24. doi: 10.1016/j.jsps.2009.12.007

PMCID: PMC3731019

Organosulfur compounds and possible mechanism of garlic in cancer

65

8.   Sina Kianoush, Mahdi Balali-Mood, Seyed Reza Mousavi, Valiollah Moradi, Mahmoud Sadeghi, Bita Dadpour, Omid Rajabi, Mohammad Taghi Shakeri. Comparison of therapeutic effects of garlic and d-Penicillamine in patients with chronic occupational lead poisoning. Basic Clin Pharmacol Toxicol. 2012 May ;110(5):476-81. Epub 2011 Dec 29. PMID: 22151785

9.   Dietary garlic and hip osteoarthritis: evidence of a protective effect and putative mechanism of action

Frances MK Williams Email author, Jane Skinner, Tim D Spector, Aedin Cassidy, Ian M Clark, Rose M Davidson and

Alex J MacGregor, BMC Musculoskeletal Disorders201011:280, DOI: 10.1186/1471-2474-11-280

10.   A γ-Glutamyl Peptide Isolated from Onion (Allium cepa L.) by Bioassay-Guided Fractionation Inhibits Resorption Activity of Osteoclasts

Herbert A. Wetli , Rudolf Brenneisen , Ingrid Tschudi , Manuela Langos , Peter Bigler , Thomas Sprang , Stefan Schürch , and Roman C. Mühlbauer

Laboratory for Phytopharmacology, Bioanalytics and Pharmacokinetics and Bone Biology Group, Department of Clinical Research, University of Bern, Murtenstrasse 35, CH-3010 Bern, Switzerland, and Department of Chemistry and Biochemistry, University of Bern, Freiestrasse 3, CH-3012 Bern, Switzerland

J. Agric. Food Chem., 2005, 53 (9), pp 3408–3414

DOI: 10.1021/jf040457i

Publication Date (Web): March 30, 2005

11.   J Diet Suppl. 2012 Dec;9(4):262-71. doi:
10.3109/19390211.2012.726703. Epub 2012 Oct 8.

The effect of garlic tablet on pro-inflammatory cytokines in
postmenopausal osteoporotic women: a randomized controlled clinical
trial.

Mozaffari-Khosravi H1, Hesabgar HA, Owlia MB, Hadinedoushan H,
Barzegar K, Fllahzadeh MH

12.   Phytomedicine. 1997 Dec;4(4):335-40. doi: 10.1016/S0944-
7113(97)80043-8.

Anti-allergic effects of aged garlic extract.

Kyo E1, Uda N, Kakimoto M, Yokoyama K, Ushijima M, Sumioka I,
Kasuga S, Itakura Y.

13.   Consumption of aqueous garlic extract leads to significant
improvement in patients with benign prostate hyperplasia and prostate
cancer

lker Durak, PhD, Erdal Yılmaz, MD, Erdinç Devrim, MD, Hakkı Perk,
MD, Murat Kaçmaz, MD

14. Jin ZY, Wu M, Han RQ, et al. Raw Garlic Consumption as a Protective Factor for Lung Cancer, a Population-Based Case-Control Study in a Chinese Population. Cancer Prevention Research. 2013.

Chapter Four – Lemon

I know what you're thinking lemons are tasty!

But lemons are actually full of amazing benefits which includes the following:

- Lemons are loaded with vitamin C

- Lemons possess a lot of fibre

- Lemons rebalance the Ph. balance in the body

- Lemons are detoxicants

- Lemons enhance the digestive process

- Lemons are strong anti-bacterial agents

- Lemon appears to help reduce uric acid deposits in joints, thus reducing joint pain

- Lemon is full of potassium which is good for high blood pressure, the brain and nervous system

- Lemons help cleanse the liver

- Lemons fight wrinkles!

- Lemons enhance sodium balance in the body

- Lemons enhance eyesight

- Lemons balance stomach acid levels thus reducing acid reflux

- Lemon help to speed up the body's metabolism which is good for weight loss

Let's take a little deeper look shall we:

Lemons are High in Vitamin C, Fibre and Help to Rebalance the Bodies Ph. Levels

Lemons don't just make tasty lemonade, for a start these apparently innocent fruit have saved the lives of many thousands of sailors who were potentially suffering from scurvy. Back in the old day's, sailors would be out at sea for months with no access to citrus fruits and would end up developing a painful, debilitating and sometimes deadly disease known as scurvy, which is actually a vitamin C deficiency. One fine day, in 1747 James Lind discovered that lemons and oranges protect the body from scurvy (thanks to the presence of vitamin C) and so lemons (which store for a long time) where added as an inventory item, for every long haul ship journey. Each day the sailors where giving a small glass of lemon water and with that the scourge of scurvy ended!

Another lesser known trait of lemons is fibre, lemons are high in fiber which is good for digestion, although most people only take lemon juice, so it's hardly likely that you will take enough to make a big difference in your health, however the ph. balancing effects of lemons are tremendously helpful. Lemons are acidic in nature but when they break down in the body they become base in nature, thus alkaline!

The ph. Chart runs from 1 to 14, 1 been most acidic, 7 been neutral (water is 7), then we move onto weak base's finishing up with 14 been the most base. I don't know much about chemistry, but as far as I am aware either very acidic or very base has the same effect, which is very caustic!

Anyway our blood stream has to maintain a ph. balance between 7.35 - 7.45. Now here is the challenge. Most of our foods today are acidic, even the healthy foods. For example rice, wheat, bread, milk, eggs, neat, fish etc…. are all acidic. So thanks to the type of diet which most of us are eating today our bodies are becoming too acidic. This encourages uric acid build up, which seems to have some effect on aches and pains and joint pain in the body, but also it forces the body to draw out minerals from the bones in an effort to maintain the blood ph. Level, which can result in bone density issues.

In nutshell if say our urine might have a uric acid level of ph. 8, for example, our blood still has to have a ph. level of 7.35 - 7.45,otherwise we would die within a few short hours, so this overly acidic Level puts a lot of pressure on our body to make the balance right, within our bloodstream. Common side effects of high acid levels in the body are aches, pain, sore joints, heaviness and lethargy and in severe cases acidosis can occur, whereby we start straining our kidneys and lungs.

Also the body is supposed to be aerobic and alkaline, so when we have an acidic diet it makes our body alkaline and when we eat too much sugar, it makes our bodies anaerobic. Now bacteria, fungus's and virus's love an acidic aerobic environment, it encourages their growth and cancer cells love an anaerobic environment as it helps their respiration process. So if you want to kill of bacteria etc. reduce sugar levels and acid levels in the body.

Also some complementary therapists suggest that an acidic/aerobic internal environment in the body, encourages the growth of cancer cells. The jury is still out on this one but definitely eating alkaline foods brings the balance back, which will make you feel more vital and less lethargic and definitely it helps to kick out virus's etc. from the body.

This is why dark leafy green vegetables and dark green juices are a great way to kick out these pathogenic invaders, as they cannot stick the alkaline environment.

The good thing about alkalising your diet is that you still get to eat cereals, meat and dairy etc. It's just that you eat some alkaline foods to bring back the balance. So you can eat all the acidic foods and drinks that you want to take, but eat dark green leafy vegetables and also good old lemons of course. This is where lemons make for a healthy alternative to dark green leafy vegetables, as most people like lemons. So next time you make up some homemade lemonade, slap yourself on the back, you've just done a good job!

Lemons as Detoxifier/ Digestive Health & Anti-Bacterial Agent

Lemons possess an amazing detoxifying quality. It's difficult to know why lemons work so well but they do. In a study carried out in Korea on 84 premenopausal women, who were split into a placebo group, control group and lemon detox group, they noted amazing changes in the lemon detox group.

The lemon detox group where put on a lemon detox for 7 days, by the end of which substantial changes had been made in insulin sensitivity and C- reactive protein (CRP) levels. Improved insulin sensitivity protects the body from the onset of diabetes, and lower C - reactive protein levels suggest improvements in cardiac health. As the lemon detox program appears to aid weight loss, fend of diabetes and heart disease! [1]

Regarding digestion lemons are high in flavonoids, which help to balance the digestive system, increasing the release of digestive juices, bile and acids.

Lemon is also a really good anti-bacterial agent. In a study on the effectiveness of citrus lemon, an essential oil, they noted that lemon had the strongest effect out of 4 essential oils on test, on 5 bacteria's Lactobacillus curvatus, L. sakei, Staphylococcus carnosus and S. xylosus, Enterobacter gergoviae and E. amnigenus. 2

Lemons are High in Potassium/Reduce Uric Acid & Cleanse the Liver

Ok another benefit of lemons is that they are high in potassium. Potassium is essential for brain health and health of the nervous system. Also, in some cases high blood pressure comes about as a result of potassium deficiency. So topping up the bodies potassium levels is always a good idea.

We already touched upon uric acid, in the section on lemons effect on ph. Levels. Basically, due to our acidic diet, the body tends to have an acidic environment. One of the things which results from this is a loss of bone density, thanks to the body sucking minerals out of the bones, in order to balance the ph. Levels in the blood, which must remain between

7.35 - 7.45. So obviously this acidic environment is bad for bone health to begin with.

But also, uric acid deposits increase in number along the joints, such as wrist elbow, knee, finger joints, foot and toe joints, shoulder joints etc. Now a lot of complementary therapists suggest that uric acid results in the onset of osteoarthritis, however, clinical research does not back this up. Osteoarthritis is an inflammatory response, which comes about because of many factors, which does not include the build-up of uric acid deposits.

This may well be the case, but in my experience I have noticed the onset of joint pain only to find it quickly dissipate within a day or two, of either taking in raw lemon juice or Apple Cider Vinegar (ACV)!

So what gives?

I'm not sure, more than likely the clinical research genuinely debunks the idea that uric acid causes osteoarthritis, but at the same time they're missing something. If I take my case for instance I don't have osteoarthritis but sometimes due to acid levels, I develop some aches and pains. Now maybe if you have something as innocent as, aches and pains or perhaps early stage osteoarthritis, taking lemon or ACV works wonders. But if you have full blown advanced osteoarthritis it probably doesn't do much good.

Probably the alkalising effects of lemons helps does slow down or perhaps even put of the inflammation process, which creates arthritis, but whatever the case it definitely works in curing joint and muscle aches and pains for many people. So definitely give it a go. If it works great and if not it's still doing your health a lot of good, in other ways.

Regarding liver cleansing and regeneration, lemon is surprisingly successful at this. In a study on the effects of citrus lemon (the essential oil which is present in lemons) on liver tissue, they found the effect to be substantial.

They noted a reduction in levels of malonialdehyde (MDA) and lipid peroxidation, while raising the levels of antioxidant enzymes catalase and superoxide dismutase (SOD). Furthermore, citrus lemon increased glutathione (GSH) levels in rats. Finally, in histopathological studies, they noted that the rats demonstrated restoration of liver function!3

Now the study was obviously carried out on rats rather than humans, but in all likelihood this substantial improvement in liver functioning, would probably also carry over to humans. So lemons will cleanse and help to regenerate the liver.

For anyone who is suffering with liver issues, it would certainly be worthwhile taking some lemon juice throughout the day. Regarding dosage, it is difficult to know for sure, but to produce a good effect on cleansing and regeneration, over the course of a day, perhaps something like 1 small lemon or half a medium sized lemon, squeezed in with water and 3 times a day, would probably be a good starting point. Also bear in mind while lemon water is tasty, always rinse your mouth out with water afterwards, otherwise a corrosive effect could take place over time!

To produce a good effect on cleansing and regeneration, over the course of a day, perhaps something like 1 small lemon or half a medium sized lemon, squeezed in with water and 3 times a day, is a good starting point!

Lemons Fight Wrinkles, Enhance the Sodium Balance, Enhance Eyesight & Speed up Metabolism

Ok first of lemons fight wrinkles. How?

Lemon juice contains citric acid which is a great antibacterial agent. The citric acid kills off the bacteria and removes dead skin, thus clearing up the skin and preventing skin damage.

It's not guaranteed to iron away your wrinkles, but it can help to prevent wrinkles some of the time and may even reduce the depth of some wrinkles. So while it sounds outrageous to say that a lemon can cure wrinkles, we have to go beyond this and realise that there are many reasons as to why we develop wrinkles in the first place.

We develop wrinkles because of gravity, which drags the skin downward, because of muscular movements behind the skin which create wear patterns, because of declining collagen, which makes the skin thinner and also because of declining skin quality due to bacteria, blocked pores and dead skin cells which degenerate the quality of skin, thus leading to wrinkle development. So this is where lemon comes in, it won't work every time, but in general, it is very good for skin quality. Although it is acidic and you will have to take care it drying out the skin, so always use moisturiser afterwards. Finally don't use bottled lemon juice rather use real lemons as they are pure lemon juice!

To use lemon juice as an exfoliator:

Cut ½ a medium sized lemon and add in ½ tsp. of sugar. Mix the two together and then rub over the skin, especially where the wrinkles are present. Clean off and then add moisturiser afterwards.

To use as an astringent:

Lemons can also be used as an astringent, whereby it clears up the pores and tightens the skin, which is a good thing as skin tends to loosen as one gets old, which does not look so good. To use it as an astringent, squeeze a lemon into a bowl and use cotton wool. Add the lemon juice onto the skin, leave for three minutes, then wash off and use moisturiser afterwards.

Lemons help sodium levels:

As for lemons helping sodium levels, the body requires sodium as an electrolyte so lemons help with his. In daily life this is probably not very important, but if you are feeling under the weather when you have a cold or a flu or a fever, there is a tendency to dehydrate and also especially if you are vomiting the body loses electrolytes. So lemon water will always help you feel better, if you take it a couple of times a day when feeling ill.

Lemons Enhance Eyesight:

Lemons are apparently good for eyesight and can even cure cataracts, or so the oral tradition goes. Apparently a lemon eye bath can cure your eyes of many conditions, including bad eyesight!

This sounds a little bit wild and there is no clinical evidence for this, but I will share here the technique of lemon eye bath and you can try it out and see if it works or not!

How to Perform a Lemon Eyebath

To perform the lemon eyebath, take one lemon and squeeze a few drops into purified water or mineral water (don't use tap water straight out of the tap – even in countries with clean tap water can still possess some dangerous amoeba's – so either use clean water or boil then cool it first!) then use an eye bath device (you can get them at the drug store or many eye cleansing products come with an eye bath), then swirl around each eye for a few seconds. Repeat this several times a week and see how it goes!

Lemon for Stomach Acidity and Weight Loss

Lemons are surprisingly good at treating stomach problems, in particular acid reflux. From an allopathic point of view, if you go to your doctor with acid reflux he will usually recommend an antacid to bring down the acid levels in the stomach. Yet if you take lemon juice (an acid) it helps.

Why so?

The popular complementary suggestion is that the acid reflux is actually a deficiency of acid in the stomach and that the painful situation is a result of intermittent spurts of acid in the stomach. So the western approach is only working on the symptom, whereas the correct approach, the complementary approach is to balance the acids, so actually adding in an

80

acid (lemon juice) does the trick. I know it sounds counterintuitive but it appears to work in many cases.

Regarding lemon juice for weight loss, this is the most famous application of lemon juice. The idea is to take lemon juice on an empty stomach in the morning, about 20 minutes before breakfast, thus making the stomach release enzymes which aid digestion. But does lemon juice really boost metabolism?

It's hard to believe so and certainly scientific research seems to be lacking in this area. I think the idea that lemons speed up metabolism might be just one of those health rumours which have no foundation, as our metabolism is largely dependent upon our genetics, our activity levels and the state of our health. Drinking lemon water won't change this!

So will drinking lemon water do anything?

As noted a couple of paragraphs ago, it will stimulate the secretion of stomach enzymes which will aid digestion but that's about it. Other than that it will help with the other benefits mentioned above such as detoxification, balancing body ph. levels etc.

How to Take Lemons

Lemon water is the most famous way to take lemons, which is very simple, you simply squeeze a lemon into water and drink it. A nice variation on this is to add in honey, which adds in taste plus honey has many benefits. Finally if you boil the water and then when it cools down a bit, add in the lemon and honey, this is ideal as boiled water has great cleansing properties.

Also lemon can be mixed in with many vegetable and fruit juices and smoothies. As a rule of thumb try to add in lemons and honey whoever possible as they are tasty and healthy!

Homemade lemonade for example, is a good way to take lemons.

Homemade Lemonade

1.   In a saucepan add in some sugar and some ½ a cup of water, stirring until the water boils and the sugar is absorbed

2.   Take 6 medium or 12 small lemons and squeeze them

3.   Mix the lemon juice with the sugar water and then fill the jug up with cold water. Add some slice of lemon to enhance the taste and either leave in the fridge or serve

4.   In a water container or jug mix in

Footnotes

1.   Lemon detox diet reduced body fat, insulin resistance, and serum hs-CRP level without hematological changes in overweight Korean women

Mi Joung Kim, Jung Hyun Hwang, Hyun Ji Ko, Hye Bock Na, Jung Hee Kim,

2.   ANTIBACTERIAL ACTIVITY OF LEMON (CITRUS LEMON L.), MANDARIN (CITRUS RETICULATA L.), GRAPEFRUIT (CITRUS PARADISI L.) AND ORANGE (CITRUS SINENSIS L.) ESSENTIAL OILS

M. VIUDA-MARTOS, Y. RUIZ-NAVAJAS, J. FERNÁNDEZ-LÓPEZ, J. PEREZ-ÁLVAREZ

DOI: 10.1111/j.1745-4565.2008.00131

3.   Investigation into Hepatoprotective Activity of Citrus limon.

Shefalee K. Bhavsar L.M. College of Pharmacy, Navarangapura, Ahmedabad, Gujarat, India, Paulomi Joshi L.M. College of Pharmacy,

Navarangapura, Ahmedabad, Gujarat, India, Mamta B. Shah L.M.
College of Pharmacy, Navarangapura, Ahmedabad, Gujarat, India &
D.D. Santani L.M. College of Pharmacy, Navarangapura, Ahmedabad,
Gujarat, India

Pages 303-311 | Accepted 05 Dec 2006, Published online: 07 Oct 2008

Section Two – Other Great Herbs

Although often used as an ingredient in tasty cakes cinnamon is an amazing herb with a plethora of great benefits. First off cinnamon is very high in calcium, manganese, iron and vitamin K. Cinnamon co is in two types, which are:

· Ceylon cinnamon

· Cassia cinnamon

Cassia cinnamon is the more popular variety of cinnamon, but the healthiest version is Ceylon cinnamon. Cinnamon comes from the cinnamomum tree and cinnamaldehyde is the primary medicinal compound found within cinnamon Just take a look:

· High in antioxidants

· High in anti-inflammatory properties

· Reduces cardiac risk

· Improves insulin sensitivity

- Reduces blood sugar levels in diabetics

- Helps brain health

- Prevents cancer

- Fights bacterial infection

- Fights viral infections

- Protects dental health/ gives fresh breath

- Can prevent /cure candida

- Benefits skin health

- Is a natural preservative/ sweetener

- Fights allergies

Antioxidants

Amongst the many benefits of cinnamaldehyde come its anti-oxidant properties. Antioxidants help to prevent free radicals, which create cellular damage and cinnamon is very high in polyphenols, which are strong antioxidants.

In a study, for example, on the antioxidant effects of cinnamon on obese diabetics, they noted a significant decrease in Plasma malondialdehyde

(MDA) and an increase in FRAP and plasma thiol (SH) levels. All of which suggest that cinnamon could reduce some of the degenerative effects of diabetes. 1 And in another study, on the antioxidant effects of the epithelial cells of the colon, they noticed a distinct improvement "cinnamon-derived food factor CA is a potent activator of the Nrf2-orchestrated antioxidant response in cultured human epithelial colon cells", which in dictates strong anti-cancerous properties of cinnamon!2

High in Anti-Inflammatory properties

Inflammation is the bodies' way of dealing with big imbalances inside the body. While inflammation is bad, the inflammation is the bodies' attempt to consolidate the problem. However, the problem with inflammation is that although it works well for a few years, eventually it results in long-term organic damage, such as heart disease, diabetes, osteoarthritis, stomach and intestine problems etc.

Atypically in the early stages inflammation produces swelling, heat, redness and pain. But inside the body many changes are taking place without our awareness. The body undergoes an inflammatory response, whereby white blood cell and immune cells are increased, along with cytokines, which help to fight infection.

While it works well in the short term, over the long-term this inflammation response results in the ravaging of the inner organs, thus resulting in diseases such as heart disease, diabetes, fatty liver disease and in some case cancer.

Inflammation usually comes about as a consequence of stress, lifestyle choices, chemicals in the environment, poor diet, lack of exercise and genetic factors. In a nutshell our modern busy lifestyle combined with processed foods, lack of exercise and stress kicks of our genetic predispositions to certain diseases!

Tests such as homoscycteine, TNF A, IL-6 and C-reactive protein (CRP) are all designed to help to identify inflammation in the body at an early stage before it becomes a problem.

But what about treating the inflammation?

Here cinnamon comes in very helpful indeed!

In one study they noted that cinnamon oil contains trans-cinnamaldhehyde, which is a strong anti-inflammatrory as it T-cadinol and α-cadinol, which also help to reduce inflammation.3

Meanwhile in another study on the effects of cloves and nutmegs, as an antioxidant in cooking, they noted that cinanamon had a 100% inhibition effect on COX-2, even after cooking, thus cinnamon even when cooked has a strong antioxidant effect.4

Cinnamon Reduces Cardiac Risk

Cinnamon produces a good effect on cardiac health, and noticeably so on diabetic patients, In a study on 60 diabetic patients (5)+9 where split into 3 groups; with dosing varying from 1, 3 or 6 grams of cinnamon per day.

After 40 days the following results where denoted:

Fasting Glucose Serum levels - Reduced by 18 -29% according to dose

Triglycerides – Reduced by 23 -30% according to dose

LDL Cholesterol – Reduced by 7 to 27% according to dose

Total cholesterol levels – Reduced by 12 to 26% according to dose

This is an amazing result and it's not the only one, as quite a few studies reveal the amazing blood sugar reducing effects of cinnamon. Cinnamon is definitely a must for diabetics and of course the reduction in various types of bad cholesterol. So definitely cinnamon is very good for cardiac health.

Improves Insulin Sensitivity/Anti-Diabetic

Insulin is a vital hormone for the cellular absorption of glucose. However, in some cases the person becomes resistant to insulin, whereby beta cells do not absorb insulin, resulting in the beta cells of the pancreas producing yet more insulin. So with insulin resistance a greater level of insulin is required, so that glucose can be absorbed.

Now insulin resistance is extremely common today, and it seems to come about as a consequence of obesity and lack of exercise. Also, excessive eating appears to upset the hormonal balance and force, as excessive amount of insulin is needed just to absorb the large amount of food. So while a definitive cause of insulin resistance has not been fully determined, probably the lack of exercise, excessive eating and obesity forces the body into working inefficiently.

Insulin resistance is extremely common and most of us probably possess some degree of insulin resistance. So having some insulin resistance is not the end of the world. However, over time it encourages pre-diabetes and pre-diabetes often leads onto to full-blown type 2 diabetes. So insulin resistance can be a slippery slope, which can lead to diabetes.

If you want to avoid insulin resistance, or reduce its severity if you have already developed insulin resistance, then it is important to eat a balanced diet. Don't eat too much processed foods, particularly foods which are very high in simple carbohydrates which force the body to push up insulin levels. So you have to give your stomach and intestines a chance to digest the backlog of food.

Taking a day or two a week and doing some intermittent fasting will help. You don't have to fast for 16 hours, just a mini fast of say 12 – 14 hours, will have a positive effect in that insulin levels will drop and as they do so growth hormone levels will raise. Increased growth hormone, will help fat loss but also it helps to rebalance the hormonal situation, as the body continually flips back and fort between an insulin fat storage state, where human growth hormone (HGH) levels are low and then periods of fasting, whereby the HGH is high and the insulin is low. This is the natural pattern and excessive eating messes this up, while some light intermittent fasting will help to rebalance this.

So for example, maybe you had your last meal at 8pm and you usually have breakfast at 8am, well occasionally hold of and have a brunch at 11am, it's that simply. Also as a final note on this, don't intermittent fast everyday, as eating many meals throughout the day is actually good for blood sugar levels, whereas if you eat say only twice a day, chances are that once again that this can result in insulin resistance, as blood sugar levels keep on fluctuating. Do a small intermittent fast from 1 to 3 days a week and other than that try and eat at least 3, meals a day!

Exercise will also help greatly and of course certain foods will help and once again this is where cinnamon comes in handy!

In a study on the effects of cinnamon on insulin sensitivity, they noted that its chromium and polyphenols promote insulin sensitivity, which in turn reduces fasting blood glucose levels.6

And in another study, they divided 22 participants into two groups and gave one group 500mg a day of aqueous extract of cinnamon and the second group where given a placebo for 12 weeks. In the cinnamon group they noted a decrease in fasting blood sugar levels, an improvement in blood pressure levels and even an increase in lean body mass(LBM) (LBM denotes how much muscle you have in your body, with age LBM levels drop and this leads onto ill health in old age)!7

Good news for diabetics - cinnamon improves insulin sensitivity 20 fold in a clinical study!

This same research paper goes on to outline how cinnamon, potentiated insulin activity by 20 times more than any other compound, which they examined, also how cinnamon reduces inflammation and how cinnamon kills of cancer cells!

Cinnamon is an amazing herb with great medicinal properties. Also, while researching this and other books I have to read a lot of clinical literature and while other herbs help to reduce fasting blood sugar levels, cinnamon in many different clinical trials, demonstrated the most significant effect on fasting blood sugar levels. As noted earlier a reduction by as much as 29% in the case of individuals who imbibed 6 grams a day!5

My advice to any diabetic is to make an effort to take various herbs such as ginger and cardamom, but also definitely take cinnamon as it is the most effective blood sugar reducing herb, which you can get your hands on!

Try to take 6 grams a day and keep it up for a least a few weeks, in order to give it a chance to work as herbs take longer to work than allopathic medication. As always I would suggest taking several grams a day, ideally 6 grams, but the most important thing is to take at least a gram or two a day and keep it up, while noting your fasting blood sugar levels regularly!

Helps Brain Health

Cinnamon is also good for brain health, in particular Alzheimer's and Parkinson's disease.

In a study on the effect of cinnamon on Alzheimer's, they noted that cinnamon "inhibits tau aggregation and filament formation", which are signs of Alzheimer's damage to the brain.8 This suggests that cinnamon may help to both prevent and even treat Alzheimer's. Cinnamon won't cure an Alzheimer's patient, but it may possibly slow down its development.

In another study on rats regarding Parkinson's disease, they noted an improvement in paralleled dopaminergic neuronal protection, in normalized striatal neurotransmitters, and also in improved motor functions in the rats.9 Now we cannot automatically presume that a herb which relieves symptoms of Parkinson's in rats will work on humans, but there is a good chance that it will.

We cannot expect to cure either Alzheimer's or Parkinson's disease, simply by eating cinnamon, but there is strong likelihood that regular imbibing of cinnamon, protects the brain from degenerative disease. Also for anyone suffering from these conditions, it is worth trying out cinnamon, for a few months, as it might improve some symptoms and perhaps slow down the rate of degeneration.

Prevents Cancer

Cancer is one of the top 10 killers, according to the World health Organization (WHO), but what exactly is cancer?

Cancers are tumors (growths), which take place when cell regeneration goes awry resulting in either benign (not harmful) and malignant (harmful) tumors. In the case of malignant tumors, they spread aggressively resulting in organ failure. In the case of benign turnouts they do not spread aggressively, but they can block essential functions. A benign tumor in the brain, for example, could easily kill!

So when we hear about cancer in the media, we tend to think of one disease, when in fact cancers are many, there is no one cancer, rather it is cell growth going awry. So we are better not to stereotype cancer, as each cancer is different from every other cancer. But the one common denominator is that cells regeneration has gone a bit mad, so any chemical or herb which can help cellular regeneration, could potentially either prevent or help to cure a cancerous growth.

In one study on cinnamon and cardamom, on swiss albino mice, they noted that both cinnamon and cardamom enhanced the levels of detoxifying enzyme (GST activity), which is a strong indicator that they can help to fight cancerous growths.10

Ok so cinnamon and cardamom are good with mice but what about humans. Well in another study, on the effects of cinnamon on human colon cancer noted that "cinnamon-derived food factor CA is a potent activator of the Nrf2-orchestrated antioxidant response in cultured human colon cells."11 What this means is that cinnamon helps to detoxify colon cells, which effectively deactivates cancer cells!

Cinnamon definitely helps to protect against cancer and might even help cancer patients to fight of the cancer, to some degree, along with regular allopathic medications.

Fights Bacterial/Fungal & Viral Infections

Cinnamon is an effective anti-bacterial agent. In a study on the effect of cinnamon on bacteri and fungi, revealed that cinnamon is quite effective at killing of the bacteria's Staphylococcus aureus, E. coli, Enterobacter aerogenes, Vibrio cholera, Vibrio parahaemolyticus, Proteus vulgaris, Pseudomonas aeruginosa and also the yeasts C. albicans, C. tropicalis, C.

97

glabrata, C. krusei and Candida and the filamentous moulds Aspergillus spp., Fusarium sp., and aslo dermatophytes (Trichophyton rubrum, T. mentagraphytes and Microsporum gypseum).12 So pretty much cinnamon fights a really wide range of bacterial infection and fungi.

Also cinnamon appears to help even bad breath13 and according to one study it appears to help tooth decay!14 In the study on bad breath, they found that participants who took cinnamon sweetened chewing gum, had less total salivary anaerobes than those who didn't. In the study on cavity microbes, they found that cinnamon oil was more effective than clove oil, at fighting tooth decaying bacteria. So next time you have a sore tooth, forget about the clove oil and rub on some cinnamon oil instead!

Skip the clove oil and use cinnamon oil on your teeth when you have toothache, as cinnamon oil is way more effective at relieving toothache!

Cinnamon also appears to be an effective anti-viral and may even have a good effect on the HIV virus. In one study they noted that cinnamon extracts, green tea and optimised elderberry, all contain flavonoids, which effectively blocked HIV -1 entry and infection into GHOST cells.15 This doesn't mean that cinnamon, green tea and optimised elderberry are going to cure HIV, but it does mean that they demonstrate very strong anti-viral properties, which may be able to have some effect at some future stage, if manipulated through pharmacology.

Fights Allergies/Cures Candida/Benefits Skin/A Natural Sweetner

Other benefits of cinnamon include its allergy fighting abilities. In a study on the effects of cinnamon on dust mite allergies, they noted that cinnamon oil had an acaricidal (poisonous to mites) and repellent effect on dust mites, thus preventing the spread of the dust mite allergy.15

Another known benefit of cinnamon is that it cures candida. Candida is a common fungal yeast formation, which is found in the intestines and also the mouth. In a study on the effectiveness of essential oils cinnamon was found to be the most effective at killing off the candida fungal infestation.16

Other common benefits, which come along with cinnamon are its use as a natural sweetener. Cinnamon possesses no calories and no sugar, but it is sweet in taste. So try out a teaspoon of cinnamon powdered next time you want a cup of tea or coffee and enjoy the zero cal taste.

Try zero calorie natural cinnamon powder as a sweetener in your tea or your coffee!

Also cinnamon with its highly antibacterial traits makes a good food preservative when cinnamon leaf extract was applied.

Finally cinnamon has some great effects on skin health. Common cinnamon skin treatments include:

Cinnamon as an Antiseptic:

Cinnamon makes a great antiseptic according to a study on the effects of 13 chemo types oils on 65 bacteria, cinnamon was found to be the most potent.17 To use cinnamon as an antiseptic, simply douse a piece of cotton wool in some cinnamon oil and dab on as necessary.

Cinnamon as a Treatment for Eczema:

One teaspoonful of cinnamon oil mixed in with one teaspoonful of honey and then dabbed onto the eczema has been known to reduce the itching sensation, although you should be careful about dabbing the skin of the face as in some cases it can sting.

Cinnamon Treatment for Acne:

One teaspoon of cinnamon oil mixed in with three teaspoons of honey, then dab them onto pimples and ideally leave it on overnight or at least for a few hours, produces relief.

Cinnamon Softens Skin:

Cinnamon is a great skin exfoliator and will also soften the skin. To exfoliate, dab a cotton ball into cinnamon extracts and dab onto the skin and leave on for two minutes before washing off. As a skin moisturizer simply dab the cotton ball or bud in cinnamon oil, lightly pad the face and then wash off.

Cinnamon Improves Skin Quality:

Cinnamon can stimulate the blood vessels of the face. Simply take 3 drops of cinnamon oil and mix in with 2 tablespoons of olive oil or petroleum jelly. Apply to fine lines and then wash off. It will improve the quality of skin in his area, taking away dead skin cells and rejuvenating cells thus reducing fine lines.

Cinnamon Nourishes the Scalp:

Our scalps are really important as hair quality relates directly to scalp quality. With age hair can become dry and also it can thin out. However, cinnamon can nourish the scalp by taking 1 teaspoon of ground cinnamon, adding in one quarter teaspoon of warm olive oil and one tablespoon of honey. Message into the scalp and leave for fifteen minutes, before washing it out using some normal shampoo. Cinnamon will exfoliate the skin of the scalp and also rejuvenate the skin cells.

How to Take Cinnamon

Cinnamon is widely available in health stores and online. You can buy cinnamon as cinnamon rolls, as a tea powder and also as an actual powder, and of course as an oil and as an extract. The most versatile form is as a powder as you can imbibe it in many different ways, such as in a tea or a juice, for instance. While cinnamon is a very tasty food product, on its own it can have a strong taste, so from the point of view of delivering 5 or 6 grams a day, possibly the power mixed in with juice or as a tea is the most efficient way to take cinnamon.

Also, from the strength point of view, while cinnamon tea can be tasty, it will lose some of its strength compared with raw unprocessed cinnamon, so with this in mind here is a homemade cinnamon tea recipe.

Cinnamon Tea Recipe

1.   Take a cinnamon stick or 1 tsp. of cinnamon powder

2.   Add to water and boil and then simmer for 10 minutes

3.   Strain and serve

4.   Alternatively to add taste you can mix in another herbal tea

5.   Yet another option is to add in honey and lemon into the mix or even boil some ginger along with the cinnamon and have cinnamon, ginger, lemon and honey tea!

Cinnamon Contraindications

Cinnamon is pretty safe. There are no major side effects, in some cases when using cinnamon for skin some people, suffer from touch dermatitis, but that's rare. As always with any skin product try it out on a small patch first before using it liberally. Other than that a lot of talk is made about how Ceylon cinnamon been superior to cassia cinnamon, but cassia cinnamon also has some benefits and in general while Ceylon is usually more potent, any cinnamon, whichever way you can get it, is going to be a great help.

So cinnamon has a wide variety of uses and usually in the 1 to 6gram mark. For general health 1 gram a day is good and for diabetics a large dose if put to 6grms will be found to be quite useful!

Take 1gram of cinnamon a day for health maintenance and 6 grams a day for relieve from chronic ill health!

Footnotes

1.Antioxidant Effects of a Cinnamon Extract in People with Impaired Fasting Glucose That Are Overweight or Obese

Anne-Marie Roussel , Isabelle Hininger, Rachida Benaraba

Research Group, Wadsworth, Ohio (T.N.Z.) , PhD & Richard A. Anderson Beltsville Human Nutrition Research Center, USDA, Beltsville, Maryland (R.A.A.)CorrespondenceRichard.Anderson@ars.usda.gov , PhD, FACN

Pages 16-21 | Received 10 May 2007, Accepted 12 Sep 2007, Published online: 14 Jun 2013

2. The Cinnamon-Derived Dietary Factor Cinnamic Aldehyde Activates the Nrf2-Dependent Antioxidant Response in Human Epithelial Colon Cells

Georg Thomas Wondrak * , Nicole F. Villeneuve, Sarah D. Lamore, Alexandra S. Bause, Tao Jiangand Donna D. Zhang

Department of Pharmacology and Toxicology, College of Pharmacy, Arizona Cancer Center, University of Arizona, Tucson, AZ 85724, USA

3.Anti-inflammatory activities of essential oils and their constituents from different provenances of indigenous cinnamon (Cinnamomum osmophloeum) leaves

Yu-Tang Tung School of Forestry and Resource Conservation, National Taiwan University, Taipei 106, Taiwan, Pei-Ling Yen School of Forestry and Resource Conservation, National Taiwan University, Taipei 106, Taiwan, Chun-Ya Lin School of Forestry and Resource Conservation, National Taiwan University, Taipei 106, Taiwan & Shang-Tzen Chang School of Forestry and Resource Conservation, National Taiwan University, Taipei 106, TaiwanCorrespondencepeter@ntu.edu.tw

Pages 1130-1136 | Received 31 Jul 2009, Accepted 03 Dec 2009, Published online: 03 Sep 2010

4.Impact of Cooking and Digestion, In Vitro, on the Antioxidant Capacity and Anti-Inflammatory Activity of Cinnamon, Clove and Nutmeg

Baker, I., Chohan, M. & Opara, E.I. Plant Foods Hum Nutr (2013) 68: 364. doi:10.1007/s11130-013-0379-4

5.Diabetes Care. 2003 Dec;26(12):3215-8.

Cinnamon improves glucose and lipids of people with type 2 diabetes.

Khan A1, Safdar M, Ali Khan MM, Khattak KN, Anderson RA.

6.Proc Nutr Soc. 2008 Feb;67(1):48-53. doi: 10.1017/S0029665108006010.

Chromium and polyphenols from cinnamon improve insulin sensitivity.

Anderson RA1.

7.J Diabetes Sci Technol. 2010 May; 4(3): 685–693.

PMCID: PMC2901047

Cinnamon: Potential Role in the Prevention of Insulin Resistance, Metabolic Syndrome, and Type 2 Diabetes

Bolin Qin, M.D., Ph.D.,1,2 Kiran S. Panickar,1 and Richard A. Anderson, Ph.D., C.N.S.1

8.J Alzheimers Dis. 2009;17(3):585-97. doi: 10.3233/JAD-2009-1083.

Cinnamon extract inhibits tau aggregation associated with Alzheimer's disease in vitro.

Peterson DW1, George RC, Scaramozzino F, LaPointe NE, Anderson RA, Graves DJ, Lew J.

J Neuroimmune Pharmacol. 2014 Sep;9(4):569-81. doi: 10.1007/s11481-014-9552-2. Epub 2014 Jun 20.

9.Cinnamon treatment upregulates neuroprotective proteins Parkin and DJ-1 and protects dopaminergic neurons in a mouse model of Parkinson's disease.

Khasnavis S1, Pahan K.

Asian Pac J Cancer Prev. 2007 Oct-Dec;8(4):578-82.

10.Inhibition of lipid peroxidation and enhancement of GST activity by cardamom and cinnamon during chemically induced colon carcinogenesis in Swiss albino mice.

Bhattacharjee S1, Rana T, Sengupta A.

11.The Cinnamon-derived Dietary Factor Cinnamic Aldehyde Activates the Nrf2-dependent Antioxidant Response in Human Epithelial Colon Cells

Georg T. Wondrak,1,a,* Nicole F. Villeneuve,1,a Sarah D. Lamore,1 Alexandra S. Bause,1 Tao Jiang,1 and Donna D. Zhang1,*

12.   Am J Chin Med. 2006;34(3):511-22.

Antimicrobial activities of cinnamon oil and cinnamaldehyde from the Chinese medicinal herb Cinnamomum cassia Blume.

Ooi LS1, Li Y, Kam SL, Wang H, Wong EY, Ooi VE.

13.   Short-term germ-killing effect of sugar-sweetened cinnamon chewing gum on salivary anaerobes associated with halitosis.

(PMID:21290983)

Zhu M , Carvalho R , Scher A , Wu CD

Department of Pediatric Dentistry, College of Dentistry, University of Illinois at Chicago, Chicago, IL, USA.

14.   Acta Biomed. 2011 Dec;82(3):197-9.

Comparative study of cinnamon oil and clove oil on some oral microbiota.

Gupta C1, Kumari A, Garg AP, Catanzaro R, Marotta F.

15.   J Zhejiang Univ Sci B. 2006 Dec; 7(12): 957–962.

Published online 2006 Nov 17. doi: 10.1631/jzus.2006.B0957

PMCID: PMC1661675

Acaricidal activities of some essential oils and their monoterpenoidal constituents against house dust mite, Dermatophagoides pteronyssinus (Acari: Pyroglyphidae)

El-Zemity Saad,†,1 Rezk Hussien,2 Farok Saher,2 and Zaitoon Ahmed2

16.   Comparison of bacteriostatic and bactericidal activity of 13 essential oils against strains with varying sensitivity to antibiotics

L. Mayaud,A. Carricajo,A. Zhiri,G. Aubert

First published: 22 August 2008

DOI: 10.1111/j.1472-765X.2008.02406.x

Chapter Six – Cardamom

We can't write about cinnamon without mentioning cardamom, as cardamom is another popular food ingredient which is famous for its effectiveness as a food additive, but just like cinnamon it's the real deal when it comes to beneficial effects. Let's take a look at its benefits:

- Helps digestion

- Helps bad breath

- Good for oral health

- Detoxifies

- High in antioxidants

- Anti-pathogen

- Fights cold and flu's

- Fights depression

- Reduces blood pressure

- Prevents blood clots

- Anti-inflammatory

- Diuretic

- Hiccup cure

Wow that's such a long list!

Helps Digestion/Bad Breath/Oral Health

Good digestion is one of the keys to good health and in today's fast paced lifestyle, often we end up eating highly processed food and eating on the run, thus reducing our body's ability to digest food efficiently. Cardamom is a great help for digestion and research backs this up. In a study on the effects of cardamom on gastric legions, they noted an increase in stomach wall mucus formation, which helped to reduce inflammation.1

If you suffer with digestion issues, the best way to take cardamom is to take one teaspoon of crushed cardamom seeds and boil in water for 10 minutes before straining and then serving.

If you suffer with digestion issues, the best way to take cardamom is to take one teaspoon of crushed cardamom seeds and boil in water for 10 minutes before straining and then serving!

110

Cardamom also has wonderful effects on bad breath and oral health. In a study on bad breath and oral hygiene they noted that cardamom was very effective at killing of Staphylococcus aurous, were studied against Streptococcus mutants, Lactobacillus acidophilus, Saccharomyces cerevisiae and Candida albinos and that cardamom is an effective treatment for cavities.2

Regarding how to take cardamom for oral health, the easiest approach is to simply take several cardamom seeds and slowly chew them, throughout your mouth before spitting them out. This will refresh your mouth, but also it will protect your teeth and gums from bacterial infection. Some toothpastes come with some cardamom extract in them but raw is beat, so try and get into the daily practice of chewing a few cardamom seeds, in the morning after brushing your teeth and the evening before going to bed!

Chew cardamom seeds for oral health!

Cardamom for Detoxification/High in Antioxidants/Anti-Carcinogenic/Anti-Inflammatory/Anti-Pathogenic/Fights Colds and Flu's

Cardamom provides very good antioxidant and detoxification properties. In a study on the antioxidant and anti-mutagenic properties of cardamom, they noted that cardamom displayed strong antioxidant and anti-mutagenic effects.3 Chronic ill health often comes around as a consequence of oxidant activity in cells. When cells become bogged down in toxins, it reduces their ability to regenerate properly. Strong antioxidants remove these toxins and help to protect the body from developing chronic disease. Mutations in cells result in mutations in the regeneration of the cells, resulting in the development of cancer cells and possibly cancerous tumours. According to this study they note that cardamom seeds and pods can be explored as "possible chemotherapeutic agents against cancer".3

Cardamom is a "possible chemotherapeutic agents against cancer"!3

In another clinical trial they noted that cardamom displayed pronounced anti-inflammatory properties and also notable Anti-proliferative, anti-Invasive and anti-angiogenic properties. All of these conditions are found in relation to chronic ill health. So once again cardamom appears to be able to fight off chronic ill-heath and cancerous tumours!

Cardamom is also for high in antibacterial activity, having an antibacterial effect as the dose of 512µg/mL11.4, which means that cardamom is very effective at fighting bacterial infections. Also even in the case of cold's and flus' (which are virus's) cardamom has immunity boosting effects, which help to fight of the cold or flu. Cardamom is high in antioxidants, vitamins A, B and C as well as the minerals calcium, magnesium, iron and zinc.

Herbal Cold/Flu Tea

If you are suffering with either a cold or flu, cardamom tea can help to alleviate some of the symptoms.

1.   Take 4 cardamom pods, 1 cinnamon stick, 4 cloves, 4 black peppercorns and 4 slices of ginger (make an effort to crush the ginger slightly first so as to release the ginger extract).

2.   Add them to 400ml of water (enough for two cups), boil and leave to simmer for 10 minutes.

3.   Strain and serve

You make variations on this cup of tea, but the point is to try and mix in several immunity boosting herbs so as to get a synergistic effect.

Fights Depression/Lowers Blood Pressure Levels/Prevents Blood Clots

Cardamom also appears to have some benefit on enhancing mood, although this is anecdotal rather than proved clinically. But what has been proved clinically is the blood pressure lowering effects and clot prevention properties of cardamom.

In a study carried out on the blood pressure lowering effects of cardamom, they noted a significant decrease in blood pressure. The same study also demonstrated diuretic and sedative properties of cardamom5, and in another study they took 20 newly diagnosed hypertensive patients and gave them 3 grams of cardamom a day for 12 weeks. By the end of the study, they noted a significant decrease in both systolic and diastolic blood pressure levels. Also they noted a significant increase in fibrinolysis activity, by the end of week 12. 6 Fibrinolysis activity takes place when blood clots are broken down, indicating that 3 grams a day of cardamom helps to prevent blood clots from developing. This is highly significant for cardiac patients, and the elderly in general, as blood clots and strokes are a very common cause of serious sill health and death!

Cardamom helps to prevent blood clots from developing which in turn protects against strokes!

How to Take Cardamom

Cardamom is pretty flexible. It can be added into food for taste, but the cocking process will kill have most of its biota availability, so either drink cardamom tea or for oral health chew cardamom. Another option is to take cardamom as a powder which makes it easy to mix it in with juices and smoothies. In powder form it can easily be both at your nearest health food store and online at a health online retailer.

Regarding dosing we can see a significant reduction with 3 grams a day. So for maintenance take 1 gram a day, if you have a chronic health condition such as cardiovascular issues then go for 2 to 3 grams daily.

For maintenance take 1 gram of cardamom a day and for chronic ill-health take 3 grams a day!

Cardamom Contraindications

Cardamom is really safe, although in some cases liver and brain toxicity can occur, but to get to that level requires vast dudes. In clinical trials put 3 grams a day has been observe end with zero toxicity effects!

Footnotes

1.   J Ethnopharmacol. 2001 May;75(2-3):89-94.

2.   Antimicrobial Activity of Amomum subulatum and Elettaria cardamomum Against Dental Caries Causing Microorganisms

KR Aneja, Radhika Johsi

Evaluation of the gastric antiulcerogenic effect of large cardamom (fruits of Amomum subulatum Roxb).

Jafri MA1, Farah, Javed K, Singh S.

3.   .International Journal of Pharmacology 10 (8): 461-469, 2014 SSN1811-7775/ DOI: 10.3923/ijp.2014.461.469 Copywrite 2014

Antioxidant and Antimutagenic Potential of Seeds and Pods of Green Cardamom (Eletteria Cardamomum)

Asma Saeed, Bushra Sultana, Faroq Anwar, Muhammed Mushtaq, Khalid M Alkharfy, Anwarul Hassan Gilani

4.   Jazila EM, Mountassif D, Amarouch H. Antimicrobial activity of Elettaria cardamomum: Toxicity, biochemical and histological studies. Food Chemistry 104, 1560-1568, 2007. 13

5.   J Ethnopharmacol. 2008 Feb 12;115(3):463-72. Epub 2007 Oct 22.

Gut modulatory, blood pressure lowering, diuretic and sedative activities of cardamom.

Gilani AH1, Jabeen Q, Khan AU, Shah AJ.

6.   Verma S K, Jain Vartika, Katewa S S. Blood pressure lowering, fibrinolysis enhancing and antioxidant activities of Cardamom (Elettaria cardamomum). Indian Journal of Biochemistry & Biophysics. 2009 Dec; 46(6): 503-506.

Chapter Seven – Apple Cider Vinegar

Apple Cider Vinegar (ACV) is a fantastic herbal cure. It is vinegar, which comes from fermented apples and is well known for its' therapeutic effects, which includes:

- It alkalises the body

- Good for the stomach

- It's a strong Antibacterial/antimicrobial

- It's good for blood sugar regulation

- It helps weight Loss

- It's good for heart health

- Helps relieve joint pain and muscle pain

- It possesses Anti-cancerous properties

ACV Alkalises the Body

This is probably the single most important benefit of ACV. Just like lemons, Apple Cider Vinegar has an alkalising effect on the human body. This is really important because a Ph. balance has to be maintained in the human body between 7.35 - 7.45. In order to achieve this Ph. Level in the bloodstream of the body will cannibalise the minerals within our bones, as if the blood Ph. Levels fall outside of this range it will be terminal. Our present day diet is highly acidic (Ph. Levels been less than 7 are acidic) with such foods as cereals like corn and wheat been acidic; rice is acidic; milk products and all meats are acidic and of course beverages like tea and coffee are also acidic!

So what's not acidic?

Dark green leafy vegetables basically. So to balance our Ph. Levels we need to imbibe a lot of dark green leafy vegetables every day. Wheatgrass in a powder form is one good alternative to eating huge amounts of dark green leafy vegetables, as too are lemons and of course Apple Cider Vinegar.

In order to alkalise your body, simply take one tablespoon of ACV and mix into 200ml of water and then drink it. It is usually pretty bitter, but just drinks it anyway, it's good for you!

Also just like lemon water, rinse your mouth out with water afterwards as while Lemons are acidic (until they absorbed by your body at which time they become a base), ACV is a base, but base's act just like an acid (I know it all sounds a little mad, but both acids and base's are corrosive but they have different chemical properties which delineates them as separate from each other. A ph. Level of 11, for example is just as corrosive as a Ph. Level of 3!),In that they are corrosive so always rinse your mouth out afterwards so as to protect your teeth!

So why alkalise our bodies?

Well a lot of ill health comes about as a consequence of a body which is too acidic. For a start it results in aches and pains, and some people feel that it is associated with such conditions as gout and osteoarthritis. Now scientific research does not back this up, but anecdotally, I have felt aches and pains in both muscles and joints reduxe, when I consistently took ACV for a few days straight!

Other than that, chronic ill health tends to form in a body which is acidic and anaerobic. Our body's internal environment should be base and aerobic. Cancer cells and all sorts of funguses and viruses like an anaerobic and acidic environment. By making our bodies aerobic and base, it protects out health from invasions of viruses and funguses, and also it reduces the number of cancer cells.

120

When we take wheatgrass, lemons, ACV and dark green leafy vegetables, our bodies become base in nature and when we cut back on the refined sugars, our bodies go from been anaerobic to aerobic. So really our bodies are naturally hermetically sealed by the body been both base and aerobic in nature, which is nature's way of protecting us from the spread of infections and also of cancer cells. Every person on the planet has some rogue cells (cancer cells), but when the numbers become very large they become cancerous tumours. From a western point of view tumours are seen as mutations and irregularities, whereas a lot of complementary therapists believe that cancer cells are the body's way of isolating an incompatible inner state and that only when the body's ability to counter it, do the imbalances goes out of control and cancerous tumours evolve. While I cannot scientifically endorse this, it is a viable theory and we shouldn't just throw it out without thinking about it.

Certainly the rate of cancers has increased exponentially over the last 100 years. I believe that the cause of cancers is:

A). Environmental factors such as poisons in the food chain and the general environment

B). Dietary imbalances which upset the body's natural balance and inner harmony

C). Stressful lifestyle

D) Genetics

So simply put, a mixture of poisons in the environment combined with dietary imbalances and life stress all set off our genetic predisposition, which in some cases will result in certain cancers and in other cases maybe different types of chronic ill health.

Another consideration of course is inflammation within the body, which is a clinical sign of damage occurring and which over time results in organic damage usually to the cardiovascular system, although it can also be pointed towards damage to the other internal organs such as kidney and liver as well.

Now inflammation simply means that some tissues in the body are getting inflamed but why? According to allopathic science inflammation is simply a clinical sign, but if we look at little deeper, once gain it appears that inflammation is the bodies way of cordoning off a bunch dysfunctional cells or tissues, from upsetting the homeostasis within the body, but over time this short-term solution itself results in long-term health damage!

The human body won't think twice about delivering a short term solution, which over time becomes a long-term problem. Cortisol release is a clinically proven example of this. When we train too hard in the gym, for example, our body presumes this is a life threat and cortisol is released. Now cortisol raises the levels of adrenaline, which helps us to deal with big life challenging traumas such as car accidents etc. But it can also be kicked off by life stress and over exercising, for example. So this is a clear example of the body coming up with a short-term reaction, which over a long period of time becomes detrimental to health.

Too much stress raises cortisol levels which in turn burns out the body over time!

So back to ACV, its alkalising action appears to help maintain a healthy internal environment within the body. The points which I have raised above, as of yet, cannot be clinically proven and it is possible that these complementary theories of ill health coming about due to long-term imbalances, whereby the body tries to protect itself but in the end it gets sick may not be accurate, but then again maybe they are closer to the real truth of the matter. Either way ACV definitely balances the whole Ph. Levels, so this is a strong enough reason to take Apple Cider Vinegar, and chances are that ACV may well help to protect the body from various chronic diseases as well!

ACV is Good for the Stomach

Apple Cider Vinegar is good for stomach aches, heartburn and digestion. Scientific research is a little vague on this because the theory behind ACV helping stomach acidity problems runs contrary to allopathic medical theory; hence it's not actively researched very much. But here is the complementary point of view; most stomach problems come about not from too much stomach acid but rather they come about from an imbalance of stomach acidity levels. The common allopathic response to heartburn for instance, is to take an antacid, to reduce acidity and it does work on the symptom. But from the complementary medical point of view, low acidity levels due to an internal deficiency within the body, results in sporadic spikes in acid which results in heartburn. The antacid will cure the surge of acid, but it won't cure the deficiency and this is where allopathy loses out when compared with complementary health care, because it does not look deeply into the why behind the health problem.

From a complementary viewpoint stomach acidity is a consequence of acid deficiency and not excess acid!

So from a complementary health point of view, ACV which is a base (but obviously like an acid it is corrosive) so when imbibed into the stomach, it helps to make the stomach work in a more acidic basis. So this helps to reduce heartburn and of course a more stable acidic balance within the stomach helps to aid digestion.

Furthermore ACV is high in malic acid and malic acid has been found to help balance the ph. Levels in the stomach, which in turn helps to kill off unhealthy bacteria while promoting lactobacillus, which is healthy for the gastrointestinal tract.1 So taking ACV promotes the production of lactobacillus, which in turn fights fungal infections such as candida, for example.

In summary ACV promotes digestion, fights off fungal infections, reduces stomach aches and also curbs acid reflux!

ACV a Strong Antibacterial/Antimicrobial

In a study on the antibacterial effects of vinegar, on food borne bacteria, they noted that it is effective against E.Coli.2 In another study, comparing the effects of diluted vinegar on ear pain, they also noted a considerable improvement in fungal infection relief.3 In yet another study they noted that ACV to be an effective treatment for candida of the mouth.4

ACV is Good for Blood Glucose Levels

Apple Cider Vinegar has been clinically noted for its ability to reduce blood sugar levels on rats.5 Although there is very little clinical research on the effects of ACV on human diabetics, there is evidence for apple cider vinegar producing a good effect, on diabetics when a heavy meal is being eaten.6,7

Interestingly the study on the beneficial effects on vinegar in people with type two diabetes, they only noted an improvement in blood sugar levels, when the participant took the vinegar along with a high glycaemic meal. So this would suggest that it's a good idea to take any vinegar along with a high carb, high calorie meal, so it's a good thing to know this.

Apple cider vinegar if taken with a high carbohydrate meal improves insulin sensitivity, which in turn aids blood glucose levels!

What about the blood sugar lowest effects of ACV?

It's difficult to be completely objective, because there is very little scientific research on ACV and this is often the case with natural health products, because there is no money in researching natural health products. By and large health research is carried out by researchers who have the backing of either the pharmaceutical or supplement industry. Consequently it makes it difficult to be sure of how effective a natural product really is!

In the case of ACV, for example, there is tremendous anecdotal support for ACV been a cure all for many conditions including diabetes, yet on the other side scientific research is largely lacking and what research is there suggests some benefits, but certainly noting which would indicate a significant effect on blood sugar levels, other than when eating a heavy meal.

ACV Helps with Weight Loss

Apple Cider Vinegar is quite well known for its weight loss properties, but before you get overly excited about ACV and weight loss, please notes that weight loss is fairly minimal. In a study on weight loss they noted that serum triglyceride, visceral fat, body weight, BMI and waist circumference, all noticeably reduced by simply taking 30ml of ACV in 500ml of beverage every day for 12 weeks!8

All of this is great, but the high ACV group (30ml per day) only saw an average drop in bodyweight of 4.18lbs, over the course of 12 weeks. Considering that the test group where all obese, with BMI's in the 26+ range, it's not a great drop in body weight. One would expect at least a

4lb drop in body weight, within 4 weeks of regular dieting, so 4 lbs. in 12 weeks is really not that great!

I'm not dissing ACV, ACV is great and that's why I am writing about it, but there is reality factor involved in weight loss. Weight loss is largely about calories in versus calories out. If you want to lose fat you need to drop around 4000 calories per pound of fat (the classic figure of 3500 calories per pound of body fat is actually inaccurate), so if say you want to burn of 20lbs of fat then you have to burn of around 80000 plus calories in order to do so, and that's why we have to drop say 500 calories a day per day over a period of months to achieve this, it's physics!

ACV will definitely aid weight loss, as will green tea and coffee, for example, but none of these compounds will give you a ripped physique. ACV will help with weight loss but that's about it. If you want to lose weight a calorie controlled diet and exercise over a period of months (or in some times years) is the way to go!

ACV is Good for Heart Health

One thing which is well researched is the effect of ACV on heart health. Several studies have appeared quoting the cholesterol reducing effects of ACV on animals and one in particular has focused on the effects of ACV on human lipid profile. After 8 weeks on 30ml of ACV a day they noted a significant drop in LDL, triglycerides and total cholesterol levels on a group of 19 participants.9

Other than the research quoted above (9), there is very little in the way of scientific research on human subjects, but research carried out on rats and mice suggests that ACV improves cardiac health perimeters and also reduces blood pressure. In another piece of research on human subjects, they noted a slight decrease in blood pressure levels, both systolic and diastolic, while taking ACV for 12 weeks.10 The same research also suggests that there is significant evidence that ACV reduces blood glucose levels and cholesterol levels!

Overall, there is good research which suggests that taking ACV will promote heart health, blood pressure levels and cholesterol, enough to suggest that ACV is a good solid cardiac booster, but it's not a replacement for healthy diet and exercise, nor is it as powerful for heart health as herbs such as cinnamon cardamom, ginger and garlic!

Anti-Cancerous Properties/Osteoarthritis and Other Uses for ACV

First regarding cancer there has been several very interesting studies carried out on various extracts of vinegar, which demonstrates strong anti-cancerous activity with cancer cells in cancer studies, which is very suggestive as to the potency of ACV in cancer treatment.11, 12, 13, 14

Now before getting overly excited about ACV as a cancer cure, it must be remembered that cancer is a very complex set of cellular changes in the body which results in the over development of rogue cells. There is no one disease called cancer and there is no one cure. So while vinegar extracts demonstrates promise, it does not mean that taking Apple Cider Vinegar will either prevent or cure cancer. However, it would be a really good idea for everyone to take ACV everyday, as a potential preventative and certainly for anyone who has cancer, it makes sense to throw ACV into the mix, as its two tablespoons mixed in with 200ml of water, that's it, so there is nothing to lose in trying it out!

While researching this chapter I came across a lot of research on vinegar, but little on Apple Cider Vinegar. Vinegar seems to be as effective as ACV in treating many conditions, but ACV tastes a lot better, so this is probably one of the single best reasons for taking ACV, in that it's flavour when mixed with water is slightly bitter, but still it's bearable compared to other vinegars which taste awful, but from a potency point of view vinegars in general are really healthy. So try to use vinegar of any sort on your salads etc., as a way of promoting health.

ACV is famous as a cure for osteoarthritis, but there is no strong scientific research to back up this claim. On the other hand there is a lot of anecdotal evidence (from osteoarthritis sufferers) that ACV does help!

One of the challenges with ACV is that there is a lack of research on many of its health claims and research tends to follow the money. As ACV is cheap therefor the researchers don't get many sponsors to research a very cheap product. Also, the common place idea that ACV breaks down uric acid deposits, in the body and that this relieves the pain has been debunked. Osteoarthritis kicks off with an inflammation response, whereby the body fights itself resulting in inflammation of the points, which over time results in damage within the joints. Osteoarthritis is a mixture of genetics, diet and lifestyle factors and if you are genetically predetermined towards it, it is unlikely that you can be completely free of its symptoms, although you can always reduce symptoms especially at the early stages.

Osteoarthritis suffers, who feel an improvement, are probably receiving some sort of anti-inflammatory response, but as yet we don't have enough research available to know what exactly is going on. Also because ACV balances the Ph. Levels in the body, I think it helps to slow down or even hut down the inflammatory reasons, in some case at least.

I have personally experience both light joint pain and light muscles pain, in the past only to notice them disappear literally overnight once I took a glass of diluted ACV every day. This impressed the hell out of me, but then again I am not prone to osteoarthritis, but till something positive is going on here!

131

Other Great benefits of ACV

Other benefits of ACV are really numerous and they include:

- Sinus's

- Sore throats

- Skin problems

- Fruit and veggie hygienic wash

- Hair wash!

- Facial toner

- Mouth cleanser

- Cures warts

- Cures skin tags

Some of these benefits are obvious, such as it cleans your mouth, which considering its antibacterial properties, this is to be expected. Hair cleansing, yes of course because it balances the ph., Of the hair, so try out an ACV rinse, once in a while. Simply take two tablespoons of ACV and add into 500ml of water and then pour over your head, massage in and

132

leave it in place for about 20 minutes and then rinse out suing a little bit of shampoo if you like.

Improve your hair by taken an ACV head bath once a week!

For sore throats dilute ACV and gargle!

As a skin toner, dilute the ACV and dab on your face with cotton wool!

For skin problems, you can dab on some diluted ACV with cotton wool or you can mix in a cup of ACV into a batch and lie in the batch for a while, as the ACV will helps the ph. balance of the skin!

For warts again try dabbing on some ACV (not diluted) with cotton wool and dab away. A good approach to warts is to tape the cotton wool onto your hand and leave overnight!

For skin tags, like the wart approach don't dilute the ACV, rather put a piece of cotton well into ACV and dab onto the skin tag. That's; it, just leave it on!

Wart and skin tags cures are not guaranteed, but ACV has helped many people to cure them.

How to Take Apple Cider Vinegar

Apple Cider Vinegar can be easily used by diluting two tablespoons of ACV in with 200ml (half a point) of water and then drink it. Importantly after you drink the ACV do rinse out your mouth with some water, because ACV is corrosive and will damage the enamel on your teeth!

For external usage simply dilute in water and then dab it on with cotton wool.

That's about it, other than that ACV is easy to take. The hardest thing about ACV is its taste. Apple Cider Vinegar doesn't taste great, but it doesn't taste terrible easier, it's probably the tastiest vinegar on the market and if you are going to imbibe 30ml of vinegar in a single sitting, it makes sense to go for an okish tasting vinegar. So really you have to overlook the not great taste and think instead about the great health benefits of ACV!

Another consideration with Apple Cider Vinegar is quality. The ideal ACV to go for is the organic version, which is cloudy in appearance and which has a strain running through it which is called 'the mother'. The organic version contains the best array of health benefits, whereas the more processed very clear Apple Cider Vinegar is less potent. If you can get the best version go for, it but if not even regular ACV is still pretty good. As always with health products buy the best quality according to your pocket. While its ideal to have the best, sometimes the best is not available in your geographic area or its just out of your price range., So the most important thing is to take ACV everyday, even if you cannot either get or afford the best quality, at least start taking it daily.

Like all the other medicinal herbs, mentioned in this book the ideal pattern is to take it daily. Not only is ACV a terrific cure, for many health conditions but it's such a great tonic and that's why I have included it in this book. It's the sort of herbal remedy, which will act like an insurance policy with your health, but for it to work you need to take a least one glass daily.

Also for people with chronic ill health, try and take up to three glasses a day, as there are so many benefits to be had with ACV. As noted in this chapter ACV is not a cure all, it can't fix everything but taking with many other herbs as mentioned in this book, it will have a synergistic effect upon your health that I am sure of!

Take one glass of ACV a day for maintenance of health and up to 3 glasses a day to treat chronic ill-health!

For a video on apple cider vinegar and its benefits please click the link below:

Footnotes

1.   Journal of General Microbiology (1 992), 138, 25 19-2524. Printed in Great Britain 2519

Energy production from L-malic acid degradation and protection against acidic external pH in Lactobacillus plantarum CECT 220

MAR~A JOSE GARC~A, * MANUEL ZCRIGA~ and HIROSHI KOBAYASHI

2.   Antibacterial Action of Vinegar against Food-Borne Pathogenic Bacteria Including Escherichia coli O157:H7

Authors: Entani, Etsuzo; Asai, Mito; Tsujihata, Shigetomo1; Tsukamoto, Yoshinori1; Ohta, Michio2

Source: Journal of Food Protection, Number 8, August 1998, pp. 929-1086, pp. 953-959(7)

The Journal of Laryngology & Otology, Volume 1165, issue 3 March 2002, pp. 176-180

3.   Vinegar treatment in the management of granular myringitis

Hak Hyun Jung , Sung Dong Cho , Chan Ki Yoo , Hyun Ho Lim and Sung Won Chae

DOI: http://dx.doi.org/10.1258/0022215021910474

4.   Antifungal Activity of Apple Cider Vinegar on Candida Species Involved in Denture Stomatitis

Authors: Ana Carolina Loureiro Gama Mota DDS, MSc, Ricardo Dias de Castro DDS, MSc, PhD,

Julyana de Araújo Oliveira DDS

5.   Hepatoprotective and antidiabetic effects of apple cider vinegar (A Prophetic Medicine Remedy) on the liver of male rats.Source: Egyptian Journal of Hospital Medicine . Jan2016, Vol. 62, p95-104. 10p. Author(s): Abdellatif Omar, Nassar Ayoub; Ahmad Allithy, Amal Nor Edeen; El Sayed, Salah Mohamed

European Journal of Clinical Nutrition (2010) 64, 727–732; doi:10.1038/ejcn.2010.89; published online 26 May 2010

6.   Vinegar reduces postprandial hyperglycaemia in patients with type II diabetes when added to a high, but not to a low, glycaemic index meal

S Liatis1, S Grammatikou1, K-A Poulia2, D Perrea3, K Makrilakis1, E Diakoumopoulou1 and N Katsilambros1

7.   Vinegar Improves Insulin Sensitivity to a High-Carbohydrate Meal in Subjects With Insulin Resistance or Type 2 Diabetes

Carol S. Johnston, PHD, Cindy M. Kim, MS and Amanda J. Buller, MS

Diabetes Care 2004 Jan; 27(1): 281-282.
http://dx.doi.org/10.2337/diacare.27.1.281

8.   Biosci Biotechnol Biochem. 2009 Aug;73(8):1837-43. Epub 2009 Aug 7.

Vinegar intake reduces body weight, body fat mass, and serum triglyceride levels in obese Japanese subjects.

Kondo T1, Kishi M, Fushimi T, Ugajin S, Kaga T.

9.   Influence of apple cider vinegar on blood lipids

Z Beheshti, YH Chan, HS Nia, F Hajihosseini, R Nazari… - Life Sci J, 2012 - researchgate.net

10.   Kajimoto O., Ohshima Y., Tayama K., Hirata H., Nishimura A., Tsukamoto Y. Hypotensive effects of drinks containing vinegar on high normal blood pressure and mild hypertensive subjects. Journal of Nutritional Food. 2003;6:51–68.

11.   Biofactors. 2004;22(1-4):93-7.

Induction of apoptosis in human leukemia cells by naturally fermented sugar cane vinegar (kibizu) of Amami Ohshima Island.

Mimura A, Suzuki Y, Toshima Y, Yazaki S, Ohtsuki T, Ui S, Hyodoh F.

12.   J Exp Clin Cancer Res. 2004 Mar;23(1):69-75.

Extract of vinegar "Kurosu" from unpolished rice inhibits the proliferation of human cancer cells.

138

Nanda K1, Miyoshi N, Nakamura Y, Shimoji Y, Tamura Y, Nishikawa Y, Uenakai K, Kohno H, Tanaka T.

13.   Nutr Cancer. 2004;49(2):170-3.

Extract o Kurosu, a vinegar from unpolished rice, inhibits azoxymethane-induced colon carcinogenesis in male F344 rats.

Shimoji Y1, Kohno H, Nanda K, Nishikawa Y, Ohigashi H, Uenakai K, Tanaka T.

14.   Biofactors. 2004;22(1-4):103-5.

Antitumor activity of rice-shochu post-distillation slurry and vinegar produced from the post-distillation slurry via oral administration in a mouse model.

Seki T, Morimura S, Shigematsu T, Maeda H, Kida K.

Wheatgrass is fairly famous as a green super juice. Wheatgrass is simply the grass which will later grow wheat, but instead of being left to grow, when the grass reaches about 6 inches, they cut the grass and process it. Ideally you should grow your own wheatgrass at home, but this is difficult, so for most people they will go for wheatgrass which has been processed into a powder, which has less potency yet it's still pretty good.

Wheatgrass has become so popular because it is so potent. Wheatgrass has the same structure as human blood, with one change which is that instead of hemoglobin at the center of the haemoglobin protein, wheatgrass has chlorophyll. wheatgrass is a sort of super green vegetable with a huge amount of high potency nutrients encapsulated into a few grams of grass or powder.

So what are the benefits of wheatgrass?

- Alkalizes the body

- Oxygenates the body

- Anti-cancerous

- Increases red blood cell count/cleanses the blood

- Detoxifies the liver

- Helps the digestive system

- Very high in nutrients when compared to regular vegetables

- Stimulates the thyroid

- Helps weight loss

- Helps to keep bones strong

- Rejuvenates the skin

- Improves the body's healing response

- Helps blood sugar levels

- Health blood lipid profile

- Neutralizes bad breath and bad odour

- Increases athletic performance

Alkalises the Body/Oxygenises Body/Detoxification

You might have noticed by now that I keep on emphasising the importance of alkalising the body and there is a good reason behind this. As noted earlier in the chapters on lemons and Apple Cider Vinegar, that the body has to maintain a Ph. Blood level between 7.35 - 7.45, otherwise the body will going into organ failure and death will occur. So our bodies will do whatever it takes to maintain blood ph. Levels. The Ph. Levels in the saliva and urine might well be acidic, but the blood serum level Ph. Will always be in this 7.35 - 7.45 zone.

The problem with an acidic body, is that in an effort to maintain the blood serum Ph. levels., the body will cannibalise itself in an effort to maintain the blood serum ph. levels, robbing alkalising minerals from the bones and in some cases even from the kidneys. So an acidic body is going to be a body with bones which tends to be weaker, but there are actually a wide range of deficiencies which will come about from this situation which includes:

- Fatigue

- Inflammation

- Joint and muscle pain

- Allergic response

- Nasal congestion

- Asthma

- Poor quality skin and hair

- Weight gain

- In the long term possible chronic ill health

So when the body fails to remain in the alkaline region it results in an overly acidic internal environment, which is inefficient and results in the fatigue and aches and pains as noted above. In exceptionable cases acidosis can occur, whereby the body's Ph. levels can drop to a very low level which will in itself make you ill, but in most cases having an acidic body will not in itself make you ill, but it will make you feel less at ease and over time it can lead the way to various chronic forms of ill health developing.

Wheatgrass been very alkaline in nature will help to right this balance. In general dark green leafy vegetables are alkaline in nature whereas cereals such as rice, corn and wheat are acidic as is dairy and meat. Wheatgrass, lemons and Apple Cider Vinegar, if taken regularly will help to right this balance which will make you feel healthy and indeed it will protect your health against the development of many chronic illnesses.

Another nice consideration with wheatgrass is that it oxygenates the body. Wheatgrass molecules are structured almost exactly the same way as haemoglobin, with the exception that instead of iron at its centre, in wheatgrass chlorophyll is at its centre. Haemoglobin is a molecule which is found in red blood cells and its function is to take oxygen from the lungs and to transport it around the body. This oxygen helps the tissues to regenerate and any deficiencies in haemoglobin, results in deoxygenating which in severe cases can cause anaemia or in mild cases a general sense of fatigue and listlessness.

143

The suggestion is that because wheatgrass is just like haemoglobin export it has chlorophyll at its centre instead of iron, that it will boost oxygenation as haemoglobin picks up oxygen from the lungs and transports out through the tissues of the body.

 Is this really the case?

Well in a study on 32 patients, who suffered from thalassemia major (a genetic condition which results in severe anaemia), they noted that blood transfusions reduced by 25% one average (thalassemia sufferers usually need blood transfusion to bring up their red blood count) 1 So this is a big reduction in blood transfusions requirements, in anaemia patients, does strongly suggest that wheatgrass boosts blood oxygenation levels, which in turn will make you feel healthier and more vital.

The wheatgrass molecule is structured just like haemoglobin save for it has chlorophyll at its centre instead of iron – which explains why wheatgrass is so good for blood quality!

From a detoxification point if view wheatgrass is a wonderful detoxifier. It kills bacteria 2 and it is an effective antifungal 3, antiviral and antioxidant4. Add all this up and you can see just how detoxifying wheatgrass really is!

144

Wheatgrass kicks out fungal infections, bacterial infections and viruses from the body. If you take it regularly the body will begin to rebalance itself as the majority of people have fungal infections and viruses in their body, even though they might feel fine. Yet in the background fungal infections, viruses and minor bacterial infections can make your body slower and less dynamic, including feelings of fatigue, listlessness, cold like symptoms which never go away, constant tinnitus and constant rhinitis are a result of low level fungal infections and their allergic responses, viruses and bacterial infections. Take a glass of wheatgrass a day and over a period of weeks these various low level infections will eventually give away.

Take several glasses of wheatgrass a day for two or three weeks and say goodbye to fungal infections, bacterial infections and viruses!

Wheatgrass Anti-Cancer Agent

Taking into account what we have already noted regarding the alkalising properties of wheatgrass; it's antifungal, antiviral and antibacterial effects, it is pretty obvious that it probably helps fight cancer cells as well, and there is a fair amount of clinical research which backs this up.5, 6, and 7

The problem with clinical research, at this stage, is that it simply states that various compounds found within triticum aestivum (wheatgrass)

145

possess anti-cancer cell fighting potential. It's not definitive, but it is indicative of something really positive. Wheatgrass will probably not cure cancer, but it will certainly help fight it. Also if taken regularly there is a good chance that wheatgrass will both protect a lot of people from the onset of cancer, as well as reducing the severity of cancer, in some cases.

The reasoning behind this is that everyone has some degree of cancer cells (rogue cells), whereby a cell regenerates in a defective manner. However, when the number of rogue cells multiplies uncontrollably, it results in the build-up of tumours (cancercerous growths). So obviously the potent antioxidant effects of wheatgrass help to either curb this cell growth altogether, or at the very least to reduce it.

There is a popular complementary health theory of cancer growth, which suggests that a mixture of an acidic environment, within the body, combined with an anaerobic (oxygen free)state helps boost the production of these rogue cells. This Warburg hypothesis (named after Dr. Otto Heinrich Warburg) proposes that cancer cells suffer from mitochondrial malfunction, whereby the rogue cell has to live of off sugar (glycolysis) in an anaerobic/acidic environment. Acidic foods result in an acidic environment and eating highly processed foods which are laden in simple carbohydrates (which are fast releasing sugars) results in an aerobic environment in the body.

While Warburg's hypothesis has yet to be proven, there is strong anecdotal evidence to suggest that he was at least partly correct. In science we begin with a hypothesis (an idea), then move onto a theory (a viable verifiable outline of processes involved in a certain measurable activity). So as yet Warburg's hypothesis is simply an idea, and it's probably not completely correct, but the number of people who are acidic and anaerobic, due to acidic foods combined with high carb foods, has never been higher nor has the incident of cancer ever been higher!

While the actual cause of cancer is probably more complex, an acidic and anaerobic environment more than likely encourages both the onset and intensity of the tumorous growths!

As noted earlier in this book the cause of chronic ill health tends to be a mix of:

A). Genetics

B). lifestyle

C). Stress

So an acidic and anaerobic internal bodily environment is a result of lifestyle (wrong diet), but stress and genetics also play a role in who gets a tumour and how intense it will be!

Getting back to wheatgrass, it can definitely help. It alkalises the body, it kills of funguses, bacteria's and viruses and it also oxygenates the body. Form Warburg's point of view alkalinity and oxygenation should have a beneficial anticancer us effect!

Wheatgrass Increases Red Blood Cell Count/Cleanses the Blood/ Helps Digestion/ Detoxifies the Liver/ High in Nutrients

One of the reasons why wheatgrass is so effective, at preventing illness and restoring health, lies with its highly nutritious potency. Wheatgrass is high in Vitamin B12 and Vitamin E, its high in calcium, iron, magnesium and phosphorus. It also contains beta-carotene and selenium. All in all it is a very nutritious vegetable. However, there are many reports both on the internet and in health food stores that one serving a day is equivalent to 2.2lbs (1kg) of green vegetables. Well this is simply not true! This warped opinion about wheatgrass took off after an eminent scientist Charles Franklin Schnabel suggested that "fifteen pounds of wheatgrass is equal in overall nutritional value to 350 pounds of ordinary garden vegetables," but this has never been verified. Taking a shot of wheatgrass a day will do wonders for your health and it does count as a green vegetable, but it certainly should not be seen as a vegetable substitute. As always when it comes to diet, a balanced approach of healthy foods which provide a good blend of both macronutrients (protein, carbohydrates and fats) and micronutrients (vitamins, minerals and other trace elements)!

148

Looking at red blood cell count, we come back to the substantial benefits of wheatgrass, which is its power to heal and detoxify. Already in the section on alkalinity we noted the research1, which substantiates the claims that wheatgrass can increase red blood cell count. When giving to patients whom where suffering from acute anaemia, about 25% saw a significant improvement which suggests an improvement in red blood cell count, the reason being that the wheatgrass molecule is sutured like haemoglobin. Haemoglobin is found within red blood cells and it helps to transport oxygen around the body. The wheatgrass molecule is exactly similar to haemoglobin save for having chlorophyll at the centre of the molecule instead of iron, as is the case in haemoglobin. Consequently wheatgrass has often been referred to as 'green blood' because of its similarity to haemoglobin and its red blood cell boosting effects.

Looking at wheatgrass as a blood cleansing agent and liver detoxifier is quite well known and can even be backed up by cancel evidence. 8 This makes sense once we think about the similarities of wheatgrass to the haemoglobin molecule and how this appears to have a reviling effect upon the blood.

From a digestion point of view, wheatgrass is high in fructans, which are an energy source for plants. Fructans has a lot of benefits which includes:

·   Boosts the lactobacilli in the gastro intestinal tract and Bifi-dobacteria (lactobacilli and Bifi-dobacteria are the friendly gut bacteria which help in digestion as they fight of pathogens)

·   Fructans help with the reabsorption of calcium which may help to prevent or reduce osteoporosis

·   Fructans lower insulin levels in the blood

·   Fructans lower triglycerides in the blood

·   Fructans lower phospholipids in the blood

So the health boosting effects of fractals go well beyond digestion and suggest all sorts of positive impacts upon cardiovascular health and as a potential antidiuretic treatment too.9, 10

Helps Blood Lipid Levels/Diabetes

Wheatgrass is fairly famous as an all-round healing agent including diabetic symptoms and high cholesterol. But is this just anecdotal or does wheatgrass really improve cardiovascular health and diabetes?

Well quite a bit of research has been carried out in this area and the results appear quite promising. While most of the research has been carried out on mice, there is no reason to suggest that the same effect would be lacking in humans.

In one study the diabetic rats where given wheatgrass at the rate of 100mg/kg of bodyweight for a total period of days. This would equate to a 140lb adult human taking in about 6grams of wheatgrass ore day, which is a lot (an average wheatgrass sachet contains about 2.5grams...so a 6gram serving would require 2.5 sachets per day). Anyway the results were pretty positive, with a significant reduction in fasting blood glucose levels, liver glycogen levels, glycosylated haemoglobin levels and serum marker enzyme levels. Furthermore from a cardiovascular point of view serum triglycerides and total cholesterol levels where down, as where LDL (low density lipids) and VLDL (very low density lipids) plus HDL (the good cholesterol – high density lipoprotein) levels where up. This research (11) aptly demonstrates the cardiovascular and anti-diabetic properties of wheatgrass, even at low dosage when taken daily.

Just to verify that this is not simply the result of a one off study, in another study (also carried out on rats) they noted a 37.3% reduction in fasting blood glucose levels in rats, which received 50mg per day and a 51.59% decrease in fasting sugar levels, in rats which received 100mg per day!12

Now this is an amazing result, which the authors compares to that of a first level anti-diabetic medication, but do bear in mind that the rats in

151

this study weighed between 150 to 200g in bodyweight. So if we compare this with the previous study, where a rat weighing in at 200g was getting either 250mg-500mg/kg of bodyweight or in human terms it's equivalent to a 140lb adult human taking 8 to 16grams of wheatgrass a day, which is huge as in about 4 to 7 shots of wheatgrass per day!

Another consideration with this research is that they grew their own wheatgrass, which is always far more bioavailable than the sachets of wheatgrass, which have been processed. One thing to note is that wheatgrass is high in enzymes, which is really great for health, especially in people over the age of 30, as after 30 years of age enzymes start dying of, within the human body. Now we need enzymes to digest food. One way around this is to eat a lot of vegetables and fruits as they contain their own enzymes, whereas processed foods do not. So when we eat processed foods, our bodies have to supply the enzymes. So raw wheatgrass, still contains enzymes, which aid digestion and this helps not only to prevent ill health but also it promotes youthfulness, as a lot of the age related degeneration, which takes place within the body can be traced back to nutritional deficiencies.

Basically we age because of our cells inability to replicate properly (which we cannot do much about), other than diet nutritional deficiencies, lifestyle and mental outlook all affect aging! So raw wheatgrass can really help us age slow on a cellular level... however, most people take processed wheatgrass and I can understand why, as making it yourself is a bit of a challenge. It's still good to take the processed wheatgrass, but do remember that it's not as potent. To preserve the enzymes in wheatgrass, the wheatgrass should be blended in a hand blender or a special blender which rotates less than 125 per minute, which is very slow when compared with the average electrical food mixer does around 14000 rpm!

So back to the study above. It is possible that you could have very significant antidiabetic effects with wheatgrass, but to get the same benefits as this particular study would require raw wheatgrass and several shots of it per day. If you can do this then great, if not still take a shot or two a day, but don't expect should a dramatic effect. Very positive effects can often be achieved by the synergistic effect of combining in various herbs such as cinnamon, cardamom, ginger and wheatgrass for example!

Weight Loss/Stimulates the Thyroid/Improves Athletic Performance/Improves Skin Quality

Regarding improved skin quality, as a rule of thumb our skin is as healthy as our blood. If we want good quality skin then we have to look after the quality of our blood. Whereas as already noted is a wonderful blood purifier. Secondly from a Traditional Chinese Medical (TCM) perspective, where there is a skin problem always heat in the blood is present. Now many allopathic health professionals will smirk at such a concept, but just feel skin in the area of a disruption and heat will be noticed, along with itchiness and often the skin, as in psoriasis for example will be red and inflamed, all of which are signs of heat. Now

153

there are two causes here. First of all usually there are toxins in the body wreaking havoc, which wheatgrass will quickly expel and secondly yang Qi deficiency (often based upon Ying QI deficiency) will also be present. From a TCM point of view, wheatgrass leafs are ying in nature (which is nurturing), this nurturing effect will often help to balance the ying /yang imbalance which is always at the root of skin disorder and of course anything which will relieve the irritation of bad skin. Pears are another example of a cooling food, so if you want a fruit which cools the skin then look no further than the tasty pear!

Regarding thyroid function, the most common form of thyroid dysfunction is hypothyroidism (whereby the thyroid does not produce enough thyroxin resulting in a slow metabolism, weight gain, sluggishness and overall inefficiency of metabolic functioning), caused by Hashimoto's Autoimmune Syndrome, whereby the body's own immune system ends up fighting the thyroid gland and making it shut down. Fortunately adequate iron and selenium can help the thyroid gland to be working well and according to one study "Adequate selenium nutrition supports efficient thyroid hormone synthesis and metabolism and protects the thyroid gland from damage by excessive iodide exposure"13. The same study goes on to note that "Iron deficiency impairs thyroid hormone synthesis by reducing activity of home-dependent thyroid peroxidase. Iron-deficiency anaemia blunts and iron supplementation improves the efficacy of iodine supplementation. Combined selenium and iodine deficiency leads to myxedematous cretinism". In plain English iron supplementation improves iodine supplementation, on one side, while on the other side selenium protects the thyroid from an overexposure to iodine. So wheatgrass being very high in both iron and selenium helps the thyroid to function properly at all times!

This also ties in with weight loss, since a lot of people have an underactive thyroid gland, even though they don't know it, so wheatgrass will improve the functioning of the thyroid, in a great many individuals, which in turn will aid weight loss. If you are dieting and find it apparently impossible to lose weight, there are many possibilities, but one possibility could be an underactive thyroid gland. So try out wheatgrass and see if it helps. Also if your metabolism still seems to be stalled, after a period of weeks on wheatgrass, do take a blood test, as while natural methods such as wheatgrass can often correct hypothyroidism, in some case allopathic medication is required!

There is also some good evidence to suggest that wheatgrass may help athletic performance. In a study carried out in 2008 on 21 women participants and 9 male participants, they split the participants up into a control group and a wheatgrass juice and got them to imbibe a glass of wheatgrass prior to using an exercise bicycle for 20 minutes. They noted a significant increase in blood oxygenation levels during exercise and a very small increase in blood oxygenation levels after exercise, when they compared the wheatgrass group against the control group.14 Now this is a small sample group and the research was pretty limited in the scope. The researchers noted that they saw an increase in blood oxygenation, but no significant increase in performance, and also they noted no increase in oxygenation in individuals who were not exercising.

What does this mean?

Well it's difficult to draw any definitive conclusions, without further research but probably wheatgrass will increase oxygenation in individuals, who are pushing themselves hard, in exercise and that the harder they push the more oxygen is used up, as oxygen levels run low under hard cardiovascular exercise conditions.

If this be the case then wheatgrass should become more effective the higher the calibre of the athlete. A random group of 30 people cannot be said to be elite athletes, so we don't know whether this will turn out to be the case, but certainly if you are a competitive athlete it might make for an interesting exercise to take a glass of wheatgrass prior to working out!

Personally I have tried out drinking wheatgrass, prior to going to the gym and while working out lifting weights, I noticed a noticeable increase in endurance. It could be placebo effect, but definitely I find it really gives me a great energy boost, so do try it out!

How to Take Wheatgrass

The most common way to take wheatgrass is simply to mix two tablespoons of powder from a container or sachet and mix in with 200 ml of water.

The other option and this is the preferred one from the point of view of potency is raw wheatgrass, as in wheatgrass which you have grown yourself. This is a really good option if you can make it work for you because of three things:

A). Raw wheatgrass is higher in nutrients than processed wheatgrass

B). Raw wheatgrass has a greater potency than processed wheatgrass. For example, its antioxidant effects will be stronger than processed wheatgrass

C). Raw wheatgrass is high in enzymes which help to break down food. This is particularly helpful for people who are aged 30 and over, as our bodies start to lose enzymes as we age and without enzymes we receive less nutritional value, which in turn inclines the body to age faster and also make it more likely to develop chronic disease.

While there are some great organic wheatgrass products available, ultimately they have been put through a food factory, so while

157

manufactures may claim all sorts of things, really we don't know to what degree the wheatgrass has been processed. In particular even the best quality wheatgrass powder products, have had to use machinery to mince the wheatgrass. Because to use wheatgrass we have to grow the wheatgrass until it reaches a height of 6 inches, then we cut it, wash it, dry it and then we have to put it through a juicer to get the juice. In the case of processed wheatgrass, they dry out the wheatgrass and then put it through a grinding machine to make the powder.

Now here is the problem; if you juice or grind wheatgrass at any more than 125 revolutions per minute it will destroy the enzymes. For example, if you grow your own wheatgrass, you will have to juice it and at the end you will have grass coming out of your juicer and it will leave behind the wheatgrass juice. But to retain the enzymes you have to use a hand juicer as a regular juicer does around 14000 rpm. So 10 seconds in a juicer is around 2000 revolutions, which will destroy the enzymes and the enzymes really help a lot of people and in particular enzymes help older individuals. But if you hand juice wheatgrass it is a slow process like anywhere from 10 minutes to half an hour, depending upon how much grass you have and how good quality is your hand juicer. But definitely companies will process the wheatgrass in a device which grinds at thousands of rpm.

So it's great to grow your own wheatgrass. But here is the problem. Growing wheatgrass can be a challenge. If you look up You Tube, you will find lots of videos where people grow their own wheatgrass and they always make it look really easy. I can only tell you about my experience and in my experience I tried to grow wheatgrass, a few years ago, and ended up having to use 19 A4 sized trays, in order to be able to make 60ml of wheatgrass juice (30ml for me and 30ml for my wife), and it was taking me 1.5 hours a day to process it!

Now this might not be true for everybody. For a start I was growing wheatgrass in our apartment balcony, so maybe the wheatgrass was not getting enough light. Also we were living in Chennai, which is in south India and it's a very humid environment, so maybe this was having an effect. Another factor was the soil quality, which tended to be poor. So we had to have a big area to grow a small amount of grass, plus we were having problems with fungal growth destroying the leaves. Finally, the only hand juicer which I could get my hands on, was something which looked like it belonged in the 19th century and which had to be physically dismantled with a 10mm spanner, a couple of times per juicing session, in order to clear out the grass. All in all the wheatgrass produced was like rocket fuel, as soon as you took it, it blew your head off in a way that the processed stuff never could, but it was an hour and a half a day, plus two balconies filled with 19 A4 sized trays!

I'll readily admit that I'm not much of a gardener, but certainly wheatgrass can be a challenge depending upon such factors as spoil quality and climate. Also India doesn't exactly have any gardening centres, so we had no fertiliser in the beginning, although after a while I left out a 50lb bag of soil and thousands of ants lived in it for a few weeks, by which time the soil was really fertile!

So try out the homemade wheatgrass, but unless you are a gardening whizz do not expect instant success, as you will probably have to do it a few times before you get the hang of it and unless you can get some state of the art hand juicer, you will spend 30 minutes a day pulling your hair out to produce 60 ml (4 tablespoons) of wheatgrass juice, from a big bag full of wheatgrass per day!

So if you want to try it out. Here is a quick overview of how to make your own wheatgrass at home:

1.   Take the wheatgrass seeds and leave them overnight in water and hidden away from light, so as to release the enzymes in the seeds so that they will grow.

2.   Take a 16x12 inch tray, it should have some holes in the bottom to let out the water, if not take out a hammer and a screwdriver and make some holes. Then add in about 2 inches of fresh soil, ideally with some fertiliser mixed in there.

3.   Add in about 2 cups of seeds. The seeds can each be placed besides each other. As to how much trays you will need will vary upon the result, so you will have to experiment.

4.   Add a little bit of soil (just a little) over the seeds and spray some water.

5.   Everyday sprinkle some water twice a day.

6.   Ideally let the grass get some light but too much per day. Again this will vary from place to place as sunlight intensity will have an effect. Too much Sun will kill the grass and too little will encourage growth of fungus's on the leaves.

7.   After about 5 or 6 days the wheatgrass should be about 6 inches in height.

8.   Then cut the grass, wash it and juice it in a hand juicer.

9.   The final juice can be taken raw or mixed in water.

It's really very simple but there is a lot of mixed information out there, probably because everybody adjusts according to the soil quality and climate, of the region where they are living in. Ideally you should be able to get 60ml from 1 tray, which means that if you want two 30ml shots a day and the wheatgrass takes about a week to grow, that you have to have 7 trays for two people. But like I noted earlier, it took 19 trays for us to produce this 60ml a day and sometimes a whole tray would produce very little grass, or the grass would be ruined by fungal growth. Most websites won't note this, as there is a tendency of saying "hey wheatgrass is easy to grow", well it is but you need quite a bit of it in order to get a good amount of juice, and there are many factors in making wheatgrass growing, work for you.

So by all means try it, but do realise that best case scenario is about 30ml per 16x12inch tray per day. This also means that you need to soak seeds every day and plant a new batch every day and juice one tray a day for two shots. But if like me it doesn't work this way, you could end up having to make up three trays and juice three trays with a hand juicer from the agrarian age!

So while home juicing is best, this doesn't mean that the processed wheatgrass' are bad, they are down in potency and enzymes but thy still work pretty well. Also another consideration is that even home-grown wheatgrass, might not be all that potent when you compare wheatgrass made in your tray at home, versus wheatgrass which is grown in a field somewhere. The wheatgrass is only as potent as the soil in which it is raised. So how fertile is your soil at home compared to the soil in a field, where nature is working to constantly rejuvenating the soil?

As a rule of thumb wheatgrass grown in a field and hand juiced is best, next best is wheatgrass made at home and hand juiced and the final one then, is the powder stuff which you buy at the health sore. Like all other herbs mentioned in this book, do the best you can and even the cheap and cheerful health food store wheatgrass is still a lot better than no wheatgrass!

Finally considerations for wheatgrass are fibre. Wheatgrass is really fibrous, even the wheatgrass which you get at your health store may end up sending you to the bathroom pretty quickly. Wheatgrass really cleans you out and if you haven't taken it before, you might end up going to the toilet frequently, because it clears out the intestines, which is a great storehouse of toxins in the body. So when taking wheatgrass at first, you will probably end up going to the toilet frequently but this will reduce over a week or two, as the toxins are thrown out of your body. Even still wheatgrass will tend to move the bowels pretty easily, so don't take it if you are about to go out somewhere with no toilet access!

Footnotes

1.   Indian Pediatr. 2004 Jul;41(7):716-20.

Wheat grass juice reduces transfusion requirement in patients with thalassemia major: a pilot study.

Marawaha RK1, Bansal D, Kaur S, Trehan A.

2.   Catalase is the Bacteria-Derived Detoxifying Substance against Paramecia- Killing Toxin in Wheat Grass Powder Infusion

Authors: NAOMI MIZOBUCHI, KUMIO YOKOIGAWA, TERUE HARUMOTO, HIROMI FUJISAWA, YOSHIOMI TAKAGP

First published: July 2003

DOI: 10.1111/j.1550-7408.2003.tb00138.

3.   Two novel antifungal alka-2,4-dienals from Triticum aestivum

Article in Phytochemistry 21(9):2403–2404 · December 1982 with 6 Reads

DOI: 10.1016/0031-9422(82)85216-3

Phillip J. Spendley, Pauline M. Bird, Jonathan P. Ride

Department of Microbiology, The University, Birmingham, B15 2TT, U.K.Shell Research Limited, Sittingbourne Research Centre, Kent, ME9 8AG, U.K.

4.　　　Antioxidant properties of commercial soft and hard winter wheats (Triticum aestivum L.) and their milling fractions

Chandrika M. Liyana-Pathirana, Fereidoon Shahidi

First published: 14 November 2005

DOI: 10.1002/jsfa.2374

5.　　　Chemoprevention by Triticum Aestivum of Mouse Skin Carcinogenesis Induced by DMBA and Croton Oil - Association with Oxidative Status

Priyanka Arya, Madhu Kumar

Asian Pacific journal of cancer prevention: APJCP 12(1):143-8 · January 2011

6.　　　Antioxidant Profiling of Triticum aestivum (wheatgrass) and its Antiproliferative Activity In MCF-7 Breast Cancer Cell Line.

164

7.   Both Wheat (Triticum aestivum) Bran Arabinoxylans and Gut Flora-Mediated Fermentation Products Protect Human Colon Cells from Genotoxic Activities of 4-Hydroxynonenal and Hydrogen Peroxide

Michael Glei , Thomas Hofmann , Katrin Küster , Jürgen Hollmann , Meinolf G. Lindhauer , and Beatrice L. Pool-Zobel †

8.   HEPATOPROTECTIVE POTENTIAL OF YOUNG LEAVES OF TRITICUM AESTIVUM LINN. AGAINST CCl4 INDUCED HEPATOTOXICITY

Jain, G; Argal, A. International Journal of Pharmaceutical Sciences and Research 5.11 (Nov 2014): 4751-4755.

9.   Fructans: beneficial for plants and humans

Tita Ritsema , Sjef Smeekens

Molecular Plant Physiology, Utrecht University, Padualaan 8, 3584 CH Utrecht, The Netherlands

Available online 9 April 2003

10.   J Plant Physiol. 2003 Aug;160(8):843-9.

Fructans in crested wheatgrass leaves.

Chatterton NJ1, J Plant Physiol. 2003 Aug;160(8):843-9.

11.   Advances in Pharmacological Sciences

Volume 2013 (2013), Article ID 716073, 9 pages

165

Antidiabetic and Antioxidant Properties of Triticum aestivum in Streptozotocin-Induced Diabetic Rats

Yogesha Mohan, Grace Nirmala Jesuthankaraj, and Narendhirakannan Ramasamy Thangavelu

12.Hypoglycemic effect of wheatgrass juice in Alloxan induced diabetic rats

M. R. N. Shaikh, Majaz Quazi, Dr. R. Y. Nandedkar

A. R. A. College of Pharmacy,

Nagaon,

Dhule – 06.

F S J Pharma 2012/VOl 1/No.2

13Thyroid. 2002 Oct;12(10):867-78.

The impact of iron and selenium deficiencies on iodine and thyroid metabolism: biochemistry and relevance to public health.

Zimmermann MB1, Köhrle J.

14Monitoring the Oxygenation of Blood During Exercise After Ingesting Wheatgrass Juice

M Handzel, J Sibert, T Harvey, H Deshmukh, C Chambers

The Internet Journal of Alternative Medicine Volume 8 No. 1

Final Thoughts on How to take these Herbs

I hope that you have enjoyed this book and found the information to be useful. But please don't stop there, as the idea behind this book is not just to outline the potency of these everyday herbs but rather the idea is to prompt the reader to make some efforts towards integrating these simple herbs into their everyday life.

As we can see by looking at the Appendix, there are over 100 listed benefits to be had from the 8 herbs, which have been outlined in this book. The reason for focusing on 8 herbs rather than say 36 herbs, like I did in my last book Herbal Medicine, is because I wanted to outline in great detail just how useful each of these herbs could be. If I tried to do this with 36 herbs I would have ended up writing a 1000 page book!

Over the years I have learnt to use herbal medications, along with my clinical acupuncture practice, and I have often been highly impressed by the effectiveness of some of the exotic herbs, which we use with Traditional Chinese Medicine. However, I have also come to realise just how useful everyday herbs are and that's why I wrote this book. It can be a challenge, to get your hands on the more exotic Chinese herbs and also some of them are quire dangerous, unless you know what you are doing. But these herbs, such as the 4 herbs in everybody's kitchen (honey, ginger, garlic and lemon) are just so powerful and yet they are everywhere and are being eaten by everybody!

The thing to remember with these herbs is:

- Dosage

- Frequency

- Synergistic effect of combining herbs

As noted in the introduction, the reason why most herbs end up being ineffective is because the dosing and frequency is to low and also herbs are less powerful than allopathic medications, so to get a really good effect requires combining different herbs. What we are looking for is a synergistic effect.

Just take a look at clinical research quoted in this book. 89 pieces of clinical research have been quoted, and that's just the tip of the iceberg. These herbs have been scientifically proven in their effectiveness, but you have to get into the habit of taking these herbs every day and in the correct dosing levels, which is usually between 1 to 6 grams, depending upon each herb and the health conditions which you are trying to improve.

So do try out some of these herbs. They are everyday herbs and at least the first 4, are probably been used by most people on a regular basis. But they are so common that it's easy to forget to take them, and even though many people take them, they take them in too low a dose and too infrequently to be in any way effective.

Ok so taking large quantities of the 8 herbs, mentioned in this book, would be difficult to do at one go but at least try out two or three of these herbs, get into the habit of taking them and then add some others as you go. In my opinion, at the very least garlic, ginger, lemon, Apple Cider Vinegar and wheatgrass, should be taken by everybody on a daily basis. Other herbs can be added in as necessary. For a diabetic, for example, cinnamon is a must. Honey is a good tonic and it's a must for anybody who is suffering from a chest infection, while cardamom is a must for cardiac patients and anyone who is predisposed towards cancerous growths.

So the easiest course of action is to try out, for example, homemade ginger tea on a daily basis and adding some sort of garlic supplementation as well. With the homemade ginger tea, you can add lemon for flavour and honey as well, which also gives an opportunity it imbibe lemon and honey every day.

Try getting into a habit of taking ginger/honey/lemon tea every day and garlic supplementation and then after say 3 weeks, by which time it has become a habit to take this homemade ginger/honey/lemon tea, then take ACV and wheatgrass. Since ACV is so biter, a good way to take it is to make up a glass of Apple Cider Vinegar and then immediately follow it with a glass of wheatgrass, which will take away the bitter taste plus it will remove the corrosive ACV from your teeth, thus killing two birds with one stone.

This is simply a suggestion as to how to start taking these herbs. If you are diabetic, for instance, maybe you might start off with cardamom, cinnamon and ACV from day one. It doesn't really matter which way you go about it as long as you go about it!

Don't underestimate these herbs, but do use them copiously and finally remember to add in other life balancing efforts. Improving health is not about taking a pill or even a herb, rather it is a comprehensive effort to rebalance our health and this will naturally require good diet, a healthy lifestyle, exercise, stress relief techniques, positive thinking and of course herbs.

Don't expect miracles from herbs, but do use them as a resource while examining your life and making various useful changes, which in turn will help to rejuvenate your health over a period of months and years!

Thank You

I hope you have enjoyed this book and found it interesting. These herbs are very powerful and are a simple way to support you through the recovery process. But do remember they are a support so don't simply swap allopathic medications for herbs. Both allopathic and herbal formulations are simply there to assist you while you recover.

If you like this book please leave a review for it:

https://www.amazon.com/Dermot-Farrell/e/B01KSVT0ZG/ref=dp_byline_cont_ebooks_1

And for more interesting and helpful information, on every suspect of physical, mental, emotional and spiritual health, please visit my website:

http://www.healbodymindandspirit.com

Thanks once again for taking the time out to read this book.

Yours in health

Dermot Farrell

About the Author

Dermot Farrell was born and raised in Ireland. He first took an interest in mental health back in the 1990's when he studied psychoanalytic studies, hypnotherapy and clinical psychoanalytical psychotherapy. While he learned a great deal about the workings of the mind, at this time, his interest in healing encouraged him to attend classes in Traditional Chinese Medicine and Acupuncture, finally culminating in a clinical diploma in 2005.

Since then he has run a TCM (Traditional Chinese Medical) clinic for a considerable period of time and also has taken to writing about a variety of topics.

Dermot has learned, from experience, the importance of balance in the three key domains of our life, which are physical, mental emotional and spiritual well-being. His approach to healing is infinitely practical and is based upon the need to balance each of these aspects of our life, in order to regain a balanced state.

Furthermore, Dermot is interested in moving the western/eastern medical discourse forward. Believing in the virtue of both western (allopathic) and eastern (complementary) healing systems, he is continually pushing for an integrated approach to healing. As the old saying goes "doctors differ, patients die!" demonstrates the need for everyone, who is interested in health and healing, to work together towards learning more about the causes of ill-health, and the techniques of re-balancing health and reaching out in a humanistic way, so as to help patients regain their health.

As well as his interest in healing, he possesses an interest in spirituality too. In 1999 he began his meditation journey, in an Indian system of Raja Yoga, known as Sahaj Marg. With an ardent interest in spirituality as well as physical, mental and emotional healing, Dermot is presently residing in India with his wife and son.

Dermot has a website (www.healbodymindandspirit.com) where he writes articles about these topics.

Free Gifts

Bonus #1 – Grab Free Books!!!!!!!!

As a way of saying thank you for downloading this book I would like to give you two free books, which are available exclusively for my readers. The free book "Juicing for Health – 35 Juicing Recipes for Everyday Health Problems", is packed full of useful healthy juice recipes and Success Hacks - 31 Mind-Set Hacks to Increase Productivity and Career Success, is packed full of helpful mind hacks for developing a more dynamic and enjoyable lifestyle!

Please go to my blog page and sign up here:

www.healbodymindandspirit.com

You will receive the two free eBooks, plus weekly updates and even free eBooks!

Bonus#2 - Bonus Video Series

You can check out my YouTube channel, which has lots of health related videos

Please copy the following link into your browser, to access an introduction to herbal remedies video. If you then go to my channel and click playlists, you will find lots of videos on herbs for health:

http://y2u.be/rWpgVltW4dw

If you find it too awkward to type in this code, then you can also find my channel by typing in **www.healbodymindandspirit.com** into the YouTube search bar!

Appendix

At a glance list of herbal benefits

Honey
• Honey reduces respiratory irritation and coughing frequency and intensity
• It's a strong antibacterial agent
• It's a strong anti-fungal agent
• A strong antiviral
• Can help to improve blood sugar levels, which can help diabetics
• Honey is also a better sugar to take for diabetics than regular refined sugar
• It helps young children sleep
• It's good for eye health
• It's good for cuts
• It's good for burns

Ginger
• Ginger strengthens the immune system
• Ginger cures nausea
• Ginger reduces high blood pressure
• Ginger helps to reduce the severity of symptoms associated with osteoarthritis
• Ginger helps to reduce blood sugar levels in diabetics
• Ginger improves digestion
• Ginger reduces bad cholesterol
• Ginger prevents dementia
• Ginger reduces the symptoms of menstrual tension
• Ginger boosts yang energy in the body
• Ginger is a great tonic

Garlic
• Garlic reduces cold and flu symptoms
• Garlic reduces blood pressure

- Garlic reduces cholesterol levels

- Garlic helps to protect heart health

- Garlic reduces blood glucose levels

- Garlic can improve Alzheimer symptoms & Prevent the Onset of Dementia

- Garlic detoxifies the body

- Garlic can strengthen bones

- Garlic is an anti-allergen

- Garlic boosts sex hormones?

- Garlic cures cancer!

Lemons

- Lemons are loaded with vitamin C

- Lemons possess a lot of fibre

- Lemons rebalance the Ph. balance in the body

- Lemons are detoxicants

- Lemons enhance the digestive process

- Lemons are strong anti-bacterial agents

- Lemon appears to help reduce uric acid deposits in joints, thus reducing joint pain

- Lemon is full of potassium which is good for high blood pressure, the brain and nervous system

- Lemons help cleanse the liver

- Lemons fight wrinkles!

- Lemons enhance sodium balance in the body

- Lemons enhance eyesight

- Lemons balance stomach acid levels thus reducing acid reflux

- Lemon help to speed up the body's metabolism which is good for weight loss

Cinnamon

- High in antioxidants

- High in anti-inflammatory properties

- Reduces cardiac risk

- Improves insulin sensitivity

- Reduces blood sugar levels in diabetics

- Helps brain health

- Prevents cancer

- Fights bacterial infection

- Fights viral infections

- Protects dental health/ gives fresh breath

- Can prevent /cure candida

- Benefits skin health

- Is a natural preservative/ sweetener

- Fights allergies

Cardamom
• Helps digestion
• Helps bad breath
• Good for oral health
• Detoxifies
• High in antioxidants
• Anti-pathogen
• Fights cold and flu's
• Fights depression
• Reduces blood pressure
• Prevents blood clots
• Anti-inflammatory
• Diuretic
• Hiccup cure

Apple Cider Vinegar

- It alkalises the body

- Good for the stomach

- It's a strong Antibacterial/antimicrobial

- It's good for blood sugar regulation

- It helps weight Loss

- It's good for heart health

- Helps relieve joint pain and muscle pain

- It possesses Anti-cancerous properties

- Sinus's

- Sore throats

- Skin problems

- Fruit and veggie hygienic wash

- Hair wash!

- Facial toner

- Mouth cleanser

- Cures warts

- Cures skin tags

Wheatgrass

- Alkalizes the body

- Oxygenates the body

- Anti-cancerous

- Increases red blood cell count/cleanses the blood

- Detoxifies the liver

- Helps the digestive system

- Very high in nutrients when compared to regular vegetables

- Stimulates the thyroid

- Helps weight loss

- Helps to keep bones strong

- Rejuvenates the skin

- Improves the body's healing response

- Helps blood sugar levels

- Health blood lipid profile

- Neutralizes bad breath and bad odor

- Increases athletic performance

Notes

www.ingramcontent.com/pod-product-compliance
Lightning Source LLC
Chambersburg PA
CBHW060302290526
45789CB00001B/384